30 Days to Tame Type 2 Diabetes

A step-by-step daily guide to managing blood sugars with diet and exercise

Julie Cunningham, MPH, RDN, LDN, CDCES, IBCLC

Hummingbird Books

To my mom, Cathy, who tames everything for the ones she loves

What People Say

30 Days to Tame Type 2 Diabetes is a fun, upbeat guide to help you or your loved ones with Type 2 Diabetes - & even prediabetes - take control of their blood sugars. It provides practical, easy to achieve steps one can take to help better manage diabetes/prediabetes/ blood glucose &, in turn, improve one's overall health! I highly recommend it!
—Mary Friesz, PhD, RDN, CDCES

30 Days to Tame Diabetes is an invaluable resource for anyone with diabetes as well as those who want to prevent diabetes. Julie provides thorough information in a clear, friendly, approachable manner. Her step-by-step plan for improving blood sugar is sure to be a help to many.
—Anne Danahy, MS, RDN
Scottsdale, AZ

30 Days to Tame Type 2 Diabetes breaks down everything you need to know about how to manage your diabetes in simple action steps. This book is easy to read and full of lifesaving, and even money saving tips! Julie is so knowledgeable and is able to share her expertise in an easy to learn must have resource for anyone with diabetes or prediabetes. I highly recommend this valuable book! It will give you the knowledge to take action and Tame

your Type 2 Diabetes!
—Laura Krauza MS, RDN
WaistlineDietitian.com

30 Days to Tame Type 2 Diabetes is a great book for those who have been diagnosed with diabetes and feel overwhelmed at where to start to tackle this disease. It's easy to follow, practical, and covers multiple realms of health, including sleep, movement, and stress management in addition to nutrition. If you know someone with diabetes or prediabetes, I highly recommend that you introduce them to this guide!
—Lindsey Pine, MS, RDN, CLT
Tasty Balance Nutrition

Contents

Who Should Read this Book?

This book is for you if:

1. You've been diagnoses with type 2 diabetes or prediabetes.

2. You're overwhelmed, and you're not sure where to start.

3. You're worried about how diabetes will affect your long-term health.

4. You're also worried about giving up the food you like.

5. You want a clear, step-by-step plan for taking care of type 2 diabetes.

Introduction

Hello, and welcome to 30 Days to Tame Type 2 Diabetes!

I'm Julie Cunningham, a Registered Dietitian and Certified Diabetes Care and Education Specialist. Before we get started, I have a confession to make: I didn't set out with a burning desire to become a nutritionist. The truth is, I chose this career because I took an aptitude test that said I'd be good at it. (I would have also made a good librarian or a lawyer, if you're wondering.)

Secondly, I decided to major in nutrition because dietitian was on a list of careers that were predicted to explode in the decade after

I got out of college. As it turns out, diabetes has exploded, but job opportunities for dietitians have been pretty steady over the last two decades.

Early on, I learned that the thing I liked most in nutrition was helping people manage diabetes. I love that someone who has a blood sugar of 500 today can have a blood sugar of 200 tomorrow. I get a lot of satisfaction out of helping people change their long-term health, and I love that I get near-instant results with diabetes.

I've been working in diabetes care for over twenty years, and I've talked with thousands of people who feel guilty, ashamed, and confused about their diagnosis. Most people don't feel like they're getting the time and attention they need from their healthcare providers. They're told to lose weight and take medication and they walk out of their doctor's offices feeling lost and confused.

Over 4,000 people are diagnosed with diabetes in the United States every day. That's three new people being diagnosed with diabetes every minute in the US! The number of people with diabetes is climbing all over the world, and more than 90% of those people have type 2.

If you're ready to clear up your confusion about taking care of your diabetes, 30 Days to Tame Type 2 Diabetes is for you.

Here's the plan: every day for the next 30 days, I'll give you one or two very specific action items. They'll be bite-sized and manageable. If you stick with the plan and complete these very small action items, I guarantee that you'll feel tremendously better about your type 2 diabetes (or prediabetes) 30 days from now. My goal is to help you enjoy good food and good health.

Ready? Let's get started.

First Things First: Let Go of the Guilt

IN 1958, LESS THAN 1% of Americans had diabetes. Less than 1%! Today 9% of us have diabetes, and according to the CDC, it's estimated that another ⅓ of us have prediabetes. When we add the people with diabetes and the people with prediabetes together, almost half of the US population (43%) has high blood sugar. [1]

How did this happen? The short answer is, we don't exactly know how this happened.

The long answer is:

- We became more sedentary
- Our weight increased

- We had much more access to food, including fast food and snack food, than we ever did before

- Our bodies are not programmed to live in such a state of abundance with so little exercise

You're not alone. You're in the same boat with more than 100 million other people in the US who have high blood sugar, too. So, stop feeling like you've done something wrong, like you're guilty, and like your personal eating habits created your health problems.

If I'm not guilty, whose fault is it that I have diabetes, anyway?

We have a public health crisis when it comes to diabetes. Our cities are built for cars, not feet. Our restaurants compete to serve "value-sized" portions, not healthy food. Our grocery shelves are stocked with items designed to help manufacturers make a profit, not to keep us nourished. Yes, your individual eating and exercise habits affect your health, but hanging on to guilt and shame just keeps you stuck, and you can only move forward from where you are right now.

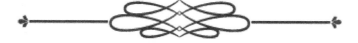

Day 1 Action Item

Write a letter to your guilt tell it goodbye!
Think of all the ways body shame and
negativity have held you back from improving
your health, and let that shame know that you
won't be listening to it anymore.

When you've finished your letter, decide
whether it's most helpful to you to keep the
letter and use it as a reminder of how far
you've come in the future, or whether you'd
like to get rid of the letter and symbolically get
rid of those feelings at the same time. Some
people find it helpful to burn the letter or float
it down the river and watch it disappear.

After you've written your letter and tucked it
away, or burned it, or floated it down the river,
your job is done. If you feel any little bit of guilt
or shame creep up, let it float down the river,
too — we don't need it anymore. I'll see you
tomorrow, and we'll get clear about where you

are with your diabetes right now, so we'll know where you want to go.

1. Centers for Disease Control and Prevention. (2021, June 15). Diabetes data and statistics. Centers for Disease Control and Prevention. Retrieved September 30, 2021, from https://www.cdc.gov/diabetes/data/index.html.

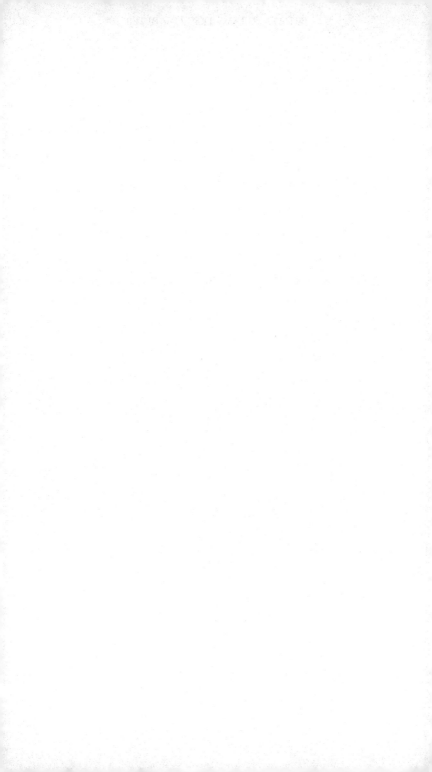

Chapter Two

Sleep and Diabetes

IF YOU NEED AN excuse to turn in early, here it is: the quality and quantity of your sleep affect your chances of developing diabetes. Studies have shown that people who report sleeping less than five hours per night are twice as likely to develop type 2 diabetes when compared to people who say they sleep seven hours or more each night. [1]

Sleep deprivation leads to higher blood sugar levels

Very short sleep duration (less than five hours a night) is linked to current and future obesity. It's also linked to increased appetite, whether or not a person's weight is considered "normal." Lack of sleep makes us want to eat more. It also makes us feel tired, which means we're likely to do as little activity as possible and to make less-than-terrific decisions about what we eat. The combination of eating more and moving less is a recipe for weight gain, and weight gain is a risk factor for type 2 diabetes.

Poor sleep leads to insulin resistance

People who are deprived of sleep have increased insulin resistance, meaning it takes more insulin for their bodies to process the carbohydrates they eat. Insulin resistance is one of the key indicators of type 2 diabetes.

Sleep apnea and diabetes

Diabetes is a risk factor for obstructive sleep apnea (OSA). People with OSA temporarily stop breathing numerous times during sleep, causing a temporary loss of oxygen to the brain and body. That causes inflammation and insulin resistance, not to mention exhaustion.

Sleep hygiene for better blood sugar control

I think "sleep hygiene" is a funny expression — you're not going to suds up your pillow before you lie down. Nevertheless, that's the medical term for having a good bedtime routine that helps you fall asleep and stay asleep. Here are the basics:

1. Go to bed at the same time every night, and wake up at the same time every morning —even on weekends.

2. Sleep in a cool, dark, relaxing room.

3. Remove all electronic devices from your bedroom, including the TV, computer, and cell phone. Stop using them at least two hours before you go to bed.

4. If you drink caffeinated beverages, stop them by lunchtime. Caffeine can stay in your system for up to 9.5 hours. (The average person eliminates caffeine in 5 hours.)

5. Avoid heavy meals and alcohol in the 2-3 hours before bed. Alcohol makes you drowsy, but it also interferes with your ability to experience deep sleep.

6. Get at least 30 minutes of exercise each day — but not in the last two hours before bed.

7. If you have trouble falling asleep or if you wake in the night and can't go back to sleep, leave your bedroom. Go to another quiet room and read the dullest book you can find using a dim light. Don't go back to bed until you actually feel sleepy. Repeat that process as needed.

8. If you have trouble sleeping at night, avoid naps. Naps seem like a great idea in the daytime, but we usually regret them about 2 a.m. Take a walk instead of a nap and you'll likely sleep better at night.

The methods above are the ones that I used several years ago to get out of a year-long rut of poor sleep. It's not easy to implement all those changes, and they didn't work overnight, but they did ultimately work for me. If you suffer from a lack of sleep, I hope they'll work for you too. If they don't, it's really important that you find a solution that does work — your health depends on it.

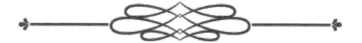

Day 2 Action Items

• Think about the quantity and the quality of your sleep.

• How many hours of sleep did you get each of the last 3 nights? Did you wake up feeling refreshed or tired? If you wake up feeling tired, follow the sleep hygiene routine above for two weeks.

• If you still wake up tired, make an appointment with your healthcare provider. Tell your provider you're struggling with your sleep, and ask if a sleep study is right for you.

---

1. Shan, Z., Ma, H., Xie, M., Yan, P., Guo, Y., Bao, W., Rong, Y., Jackson, C. L., Hu, F. B., & Liu, L. (2015). Sleep Duration and Risk of Type 2 Diabetes: A Meta-analysis of Prospective Studies. Diabetes Care, 38(3), 529–537. https://doi.org/10.2337/dc14-2073

Chapter Three

Get Ready to Move

HATE THE THOUGHT OF exercise? Actually, me too. People sometimes assume that because my job title is Registered Dietitian Nutritionist, I probably spend my weekends doing triathlons. Not so! My family likes to joke that I'm barely coordinated well enough to walk, and I'm a lot more interested in reading than sweating. The truth is, the only forms of exercise I've ever liked are walking and yoga, but...

Exercise is essential for managing type 2 diabetes

With that said, physical activity is a must for taming type 2 diabetes. (We don't have to call it exercise if you don't want — we can call it "activity" or "movement" or any other word that suits you better.)

If you already have a regular exercise routine and you get at least 150 minutes of physical activity every week (30 minutes 5 days a week, or some similar combination), you're doing great. You can ignore today's action item, you overachiever!

I have a plan for the rest of us. It's easy, so don't worry. We're going to use the American Heart Association's Beginner Walking Plan. With each new day of the Tame Type 2 series, you'll get a very small walking goal. We'll start out in just 5-minute chunks of time, so there's no need to worry that you won't be able to handle it.

What if I have physical limitations?

If walking isn't for you, that's OK. There are plenty of exercises you can do from the comfort of your home. Try a chair workout as a starting point: search the internet for "chair exercises" or "seated workout" until you find an instructor you enjoy.

How much does exercise affect my diabetes?

Everybody is different. There are no guarantees, but a thirty-minute walking session will usually lower your blood sugar somewhere between 20 and 50 points. We're going to start off slowly, so you may not see that kind of a drop in your blood sugar at first.

How can I get ready to exercise with diabetes?

1. Make sure you have shoes that fit well. They don't need to be fancy or expensive, they just need to be supportive and comfortable.

2. Consider diabetic socks, which are made for people with neuropathy (loss of sensation) in their feet. Diabetic socks are seamless so that they won't cause blisters on the feet of people who can't feel blisters forming.

3. If you're on medication or insulin, make sure your blood sugar isn't too low before you exercise. You know your body best,

but a general rule is that your blood sugar should be at least 120 before you start exercising.

4. If you tend to run low, take some glucose tabs or hard candy on your walk, in case of low blood sugar.

5. Drink plenty of water.

The absolute worst part of exercise for most people is getting out of the house and into the outside world. But...on our first day together, you let go of your guilt and shame, and today, you can take up all the space you like while you're out in the world getting the activity you need.

It's time to take care of you like you're important. Because you are.

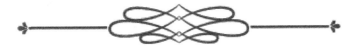

Day 3 Action Items

1. If you're not able to walk, keep looking until you find a seated exercise program

you like. Get your chair ready, and find 2 soup cans you can use for weights if needed.

2. If you're able to walk, find a comfortable pair of shoes and some good socks. Place them in the most convenient spot you can find, so you'll know exactly where they are when you need them, tomorrow.

3. Whether you're walking or doing chair exercises, get out your calendar. Choose a time of day that's convenient for you to exercise. Schedule your walk on your calendar every day for the next 28 days just like you would schedule a doctor's appointment or a meeting with a friend, and don't let anything stand in your way. **You're worth it.**

4. If you use a paper calendar, schedule your walking or chair exercise in INK.

5. From now on, if someone asks you to do something else during that time, you can honestly say, "I can't, I already have something on my calendar." Repeat that phrase out loud until you're comfortable with those words. If you haven't been taking care of yourself, saying those words

might feel foreign at first, but I promise, you'll get the hang of it.

Food & *Mood* Journal Date:_____

Time	Hunger level 1-5 before eating	What, Where, & Why I Ate	Hunger level 1-5 after eating

Chapter Four

Stress Eating

A FEW DAYS AGO, I asked a client what she thought was the biggest thing holding her back from changing her health. Her answer? Stress eating. She said she was afraid she'd be unable to cope with stress if she couldn't turn to food for comfort. She wouldn't know what to do without using food to soothe her emotions.

Feel-good hormones: Serotonin and dopamine

It's normal and natural to reach for things that make us feel better, even temporarily, when we're under stress. We actually get a tiny little bit of the feel-good hormones called serotonin and dopamine when we eat, and those hormones do improve our moods. Those little doses of serotonin and dopamine are the reasons why eating makes us feel better when we're stressed out.

Stress eating and diabetes

Stress eating not only makes weight management difficult, it also affects your blood sugar. Depending on the foods you choose to eat when you're stressed, you may take in a lot more carbohydrates than you need, sending your blood sugar skyrocketing. If you're a stress-eater with diabetes, it's super important to find another way to cope.

What causes your stress eating?

Right now, you may not realize that you reach for food to soothe your feelings. Or, you may be acutely aware that you're a stress eater, but you just don't have the tools you need to find another way. You might already know the things that make you reach for a bag of chips or a chocolate muffin, or you might not be aware of your stress eating triggers at all.

How to stop stress eating

1. The first step to stopping the stress eating cycle is to notice when it's happening, during the moment. To help clients with this, I use a tool called a Food and Mood Journal. It's a simple tool to help you notice why you eat when you eat.

2. Think of your appetite as a gas gauge. There's an E for empty on one side, and an F for full on the other side. Think of your body's "hunger gauge" on a scale of 1 to 5, with 1 being completely empty, and 5 being overstuffed.

3. Imagine feeding yourself so that you never got below a 2, and you never got past a 4. That would be ideal — you'd never feel starved or stuffed. If you've been using food to cope with your feelings for a long time, it might take a while to get there. That's OK. You're taking tiny steps toward better blood sugars every day.

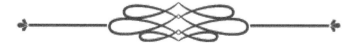

Day 4 Action Items

1. Get a simple notebook and create 3 columns on your page. Label the left-hand column "Hunger/fullness before eating." Label the middle column "What I ate, where I was, and how I felt." Label the right-hand column "Hunger/fullness after eating." As you move through the week, you'll use a new page for each day, and we'll call this your "Food and Mood Journal."

2. Record your hunger level from 1-5 before and after each time you eat.

3. Write down the foods you eat, where you're eating them, and how you're feeling.

4. Next week, after you've got a full week recorded, you'll take a look at your journal to find clues to your stress eating triggers.

5. Walk at an easy pace for 10 minutes, stretch for 2 minutes, and then walk at an easy pace for another 5-10 minutes after you stretch.

Chapter Five

Stress Management

HAVE YOU EVER HEARD of "flight or fight syndrome?" It explains a lot about stress and diabetes. Flight or fight syndrome was first described by an American physiologist by the name of Walter Cannon in the 1920s. Walter Cannon figured out that when we're stressed, our bodies prepare to fight with or flee from whatever is stressing us out. We get a release of hormones into our bloodstream to help us do that.

The two main hormones associated with stress and diabetes are:

- Adrenaline
- Cortisol

You may have heard of adrenaline and cortisol before. Adrenaline is like a chemical signal that tells your body to speed things up — that includes your heart rate and your blood pressure.

Cortisol tells your body that you need lots of energy to fight with or flee from this big scary thing that's coming at you. Cortisol signals the body to dump sugar into the bloodstream.

An example of fight or flight syndrome

Imagine that you're living on a farm in the 1800s. You're peacefully planting your fields when you come this close to stepping on a nest of rattlesnakes. (Sorry, snake lovers... bear with me!) Lucky for you, your flight or fight syndrome kicks in, and in the blink of an eye, you pull back your foot, pivot, and run in the other direction before the rattlesnake sinks his fangs into your flesh.

In this case, fight or flight syndrome worked perfectly. Your body got the energy it needed to quickly flee from something dangerous.

Fight or flight syndrome today

I don't know about you, but I don't spend any time planting fields. There is an occasional bear spotted in my neighborhood, but despite my daily walk, I've never actually seen one myself. Thankfully, I can't remember the last time that I needed to physically run from or fight with something.

The things that stress us out today are less physical and more mental. We're stressed out by deadlines, bills, traffic, and lots of other things that we can't physically fight with or flee from.

But...our bodies don't know that. When we get a big ugly credit card bill in the mail and it feels stressful, we still get a release of adrenaline and cortisol in our bloodstream. Those hormones still raise our blood pressure and our heart rate as well as our blood sugar, even if we're just standing by the mailbox or sitting on the couch.

Mental stress and diabetes, and how to manage it

Now that you know how stress affects your blood sugar, you need a plan to manage it. You need a way to lower your overall level of stress as well as a way to cope with stress at the moment when it pops up in your everyday life.

Immediate ways to lower stress anywhere:

1. **Use a "breath" prayer or meditation.** When you breathe in, imagine something good coming into your body, such as "peace". Take in a full breath through your nose while you say the word "peace" inside your head. Hold onto that thought and that breath for several beats, and then breath out through your nose, emptying your breath and mentally imagining something negative leaving your body, such as "tension". Repeat that process ten times or more, until you feel relaxed.

2. **Progressive muscle relaxation.** Mentally scan your body from top to bottom, tensing up every muscle you can find, and then consciously relaxing it. This works

best lying down, but you can also do this in a chair if you need to.

3. **"Square" breathing.** Breathe in for the count of four, then hold your breath for the count of four, then breathe out to the count of four, then hold your breath again to the count of four. Repeat as many times as needed.

Longer-term ways to lower stress:

1. Sleep. If you're not getting enough good quality sleep, your stress levels will go up. Sleep is not a luxury, it's a necessity.

2. Physical activity: get at least 30 minutes a day, and preferably more. You don't have to run a marathon, but you might be surprised what a regular walk outdoors will do to elevate your mood.

3. Yoga, tai chi, and meditation are excellent ways to reduce stress.

4. Develop a hobby that absorbs your focus. It really doesn't matter what the hobby is, just that it requires your concentration so you can't think about your problems while you think about the hobby.

5. Professional mental health counseling. Many people with diabetes suffer from depression due to the strain of living with a chronic illness. There's no shame in getting help from a trained professional; in fact, it's the smart thing to do.

The bottom line about stress and diabetes

Your brain doesn't know the difference between a big ugly rattlesnake and a big ugly credit card bill. Your body will release the same stress hormones in any situation that upsets you. That's great for rattlesnakes, but not so great for the rest of what ails you, as my grandparents would have said. So, it's up to you to make a plan to manage your stress in order to keep your blood sugar levels where you want them.

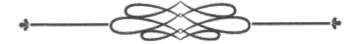

Day 5 Action Items

1. Assess your own stress level. How well do you manage stress?

2. Choose one short-term and one long-term method of coping with stress and practice them today.

3. Walk at an easy pace for 10-15 minutes.

Chapter Six

Your Blood Sugars and A1c

Blood Sugars: What's normal, and what's not?

Fasting blood sugars (first thing in the morning, before any food or drink):

• A fasting blood sugar of less than 100 is considered ideal.

• A fasting blood sugar between 101 and 125 is considered prediabetic.

• A fasting blood sugar of 126 on two different days is enough for a physician to diagnose a person with diabetes.

Post-meal blood sugars (1-2 hours after the start of a meal):

- A post-meal blood sugar of less than 140 mg/dl is typical of a person without diabetes.

- A post-meal blood sugar of less than 180 mg/dl is the American Diabetes Association's recommended goal for people with diabetes.

Your A1c

Before we talk about your A1c, let's talk about donuts. I know I'm odd, but I don't really like them. They smell great, but the taste never measures up to the smell for me. Lest you think I'm one of those people who just doesn't like sweets, rest assured that there are days when I'd drive 20 miles for a chocolate bar!

What I do like about donuts is using them to explain hemoglobin A1c, and that's what I'm going to do now.

Diabetes and hemoglobin A1c

Hemoglobin is the medical word for "red blood cells." The "A1c" means "glycated", or covered in sugar. To put it simply, the hemoglobin A1c test measures the percentage of your red blood cells that are sugar-coated.

Every day, your body makes new red blood cells, and every day, old blood cells outlive their usefulness and get destroyed. The lifetime of a red blood cell inside your body is about 3 months.

Your red blood cells are donut-shaped. Think of them as plain, unglazed donuts. If you have a healthy amount of sugar in your bloodstream, just a few of your red blood cells will become glazed with sugar.

As your blood sugar rises, more and more of your red blood cells will become glycated, that is, more and more of your "donuts" will become "glazed."

Think about a box filled with a dozen donuts. Imagine that a person with well-managed diabetes has only one glazed donut in her box, while another person with poorly controlled diabetes might have 2 or 3 glazed donuts in his box.

Why do I need to control my A1c?

Those glazed donuts, or sugar-coated red blood cells, damage the tiniest of blood vessels in your body, the ones in your eyes, your kidneys, and your hands and feet — all the places where people with diabetes have complications.

What's a normal hemoglobin A1c?

- A person without diabetes will have an A1c of 5.6% or less.

- The prediabetic range is 5.7-6.4%,

- An A1c of 6.5% or more is high enough to diagnose diabetes.

- For people with diabetes, the American Diabetes Association's recommended goal is to keep the A1c under 7%. This helps prevent long-term damage to the eyes, kidneys, and other tissues.

How often should my doctor check my A1c?

Getting a new A1c test every couple of weeks isn't useful, because most of the same red blood cells are still floating around in your bloodstream, and once they become sugar-coated, they stay that way. Remember when we said that each red blood cell lives in your body for about 3 months? That's why your doctor doesn't run this test more often than every 3-6 months. If you have diabetes and your A1c is good, your doctor will probably wait 6 months or more in between tests.

How can I lower my A1c?

The best way to lower your A1c is to lower your daily blood sugar readings. If your daily blood sugar levels are good, your A1c will be good, too. (You'll only have too many glazed donuts in your box if you have too much sugar in your bloodstream most of the time.) So, you can't change your A1c today, but you can start to change your blood sugar today, and that will change your A1c in the long run.

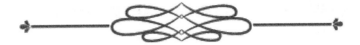

Day 6 Action Items

1. Do you know your most recent A1c? If so, was it under 7?

2. If you don't know your most recent A1c, or if you haven't had an A1c test in more than six months, or if your last A1c was above 7, call your health care provider to schedule an A1c test.

Walk at an easy pace for 15-20 minutes, stretch for 2 minutes.

Chapter Seven

Macronutrients

COUNTING "MACROS" IS ALL the rage in the weight loss industry these days, but what about macronutrients and diabetes? Today's topic is dietary macros and how they affect your blood sugar.

What are macronutrients?

Macro is an abbreviation for the word macronutrients. The word macro means "large." A macronutrient is an energy-containing component of food. Our bodies use macros for fuel.

In contrast, micronutrients ("small" nutrients) are necessary components of food that don't give us calories when we eat them, like vitamins and minerals.

Three types of macros

• Protein: nutrients that help us build and maintain our muscles. Protein can be used as fuel if needed.

• Fat: nutrients that help us insulate and protect our bodies, and can also be used as fuel.

• Carbohydrate: nutrients that are primarily used as fuel for muscles and brain cells.

Macronutrients and diabetes: Which macros affect blood sugar?

Neither fat nor protein affects your blood sugar in any significant way. Carbohydrate is the macronutrient that's most important for managing diabetes.

Carbohydrates are chains of sugar molecules. When we digest them, our blood sugar increases. There are two main types of carbohydrates:

- Simple carbohydrates are broken down quickly in our digestive tracts. These foods lack fiber. Simple carbs are naturally found in foods like milk and fruit. Sugar-sweetened foods like cakes, pies, and soft drinks are loaded with simple carbohydrates.

- Complex carbohydrates are long chains of sugar molecules. Complex carbs are broken down into glucose (sugar) molecules just like simple carbs are, but they usually have added fiber, which slows our digestion and means that our blood sugar levels don't rise as quickly when we eat them.

When it comes to macros and diabetes, complex carbs are the best choice for keeping blood sugar in range.

Examples of simple carbohydrates

- Milk
- Yogurt
- Juice
- Honey
- Candy

Examples of complex carbohydrates

- Vegetables

- Beans

- Lentils

- Whole-grain bread

- Brown rice

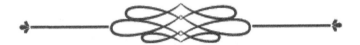

Day 7 Action Items

1. Decide on just one simple carb that you could eliminate from your diet. For example, if you usually drink 3 regular sodas a day, you might decide to cut back to 2 regular soft drinks and drink a diet soda or water instead of the third. Make your goal something you know you can realistically accomplish — don't set yourself up for failure by choosing a goal you're not likely to meet. Write down your goal, and make a plan for how you'll

accomplish it. Do you need to get rid of your sugar bin, or take a different route to work so you won't drive by your favorite fast-food restaurant?

2. No walking today! Take a well-deserved rest.

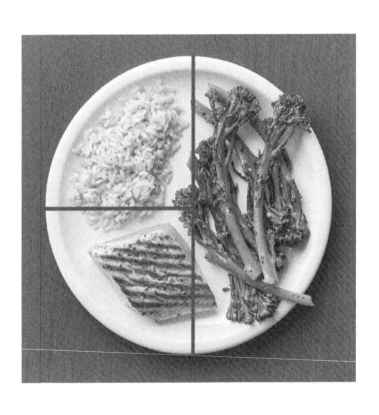

Chapter Eight

The Plate Method

The plate method

HAVE YOU EVER HEARD of the plate method? It's one of the simplest ways to portion out your food without needing to break out a food scale or even your measuring cups. If you like to keep things simple, the plate method can help you balance your blood sugar and manage your diabetes without a lot of fuss.

What is the plate method?

The plate method is a simple way of sectioning your plate that helps you understand how much of each type of macronutrient you need at each meal, without measuring.

How to use the plate method to manage eating with diabetes

To use the plate method, follow these steps:

1. Find a plate that measures nine inches across. That's the same size as a standard paper plate. If you have older dishes, they may be just the right size. Newer dishes sometimes measure as much as twelve inches in diameter. That's no good — if you put a reasonable amount of food on a very large plate, the plate looks empty. You'll probably feel like you're not getting enough to eat because your eyes will tell you that your plate is bare. So, if you have larger dinner plates at home, try using a salad plate for your meals.

2. Imagine a line down the center of your plate.

3. Divide the right-hand side of your plate in half with another imaginary line.

4. Your plate is now ready to help you perfect your portion sizes.

5. The larger (half-sized) section of your plate is where your non-starchy vegetables belong. Fill up that half your plate with these goodies from the garden as many times as you like. They won't raise your blood sugar and they will help you feel full.

6. The other half of your plate (the size divided into quarters) is where your protein and carbohydrate foods belong.

7. Eat a serving of protein about the size of a deck of cards two to three times a day.

8. Eat a serving of starchy (carb-containing) foods with each meal. The higher the fiber content of your carbohydrate foods, the better.

9. Off to the side of your plate, add a serving of fruit and a serving of milk if you like.

Each serving of starch, milk, and fruit has about 15 grams of carbohydrate, so if you use the plate method, you'll end up with about 45 grams of carbohydrate per meal. This is a reasonable amount for most people, but it's just a ballpark figure. Your personal needs may vary according to your age, gender, and activity level.

The plate method and your diabetes medications

If you take medications that have a potential side effect of low blood sugar, including insulin, pay close attention to your blood sugars. If you've been eating significantly more (or less) than 45 grams of carbohydrate per meal, your blood sugars may be very different from your normal levels, and your food or medication may need to be adjusted. A Registered Dietitian Nutritionist who specializes in diabetes can help you with this.

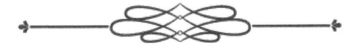

Day 8 Action Items

1. Measure the plates you normally use at home.

2. If your plate is wider than nine inches across, find a smaller plate. It could be a salad plate or a paper plate. There are also divided plates made for people with diabetes. I particularly like the Uba plate because it can pass for regular dinnerware and doesn't look like it's made for a preschooler. You can see the Uba plate on the resources page of my website: https://www.juliecunninghamrd.com/resources

3. Each time you eat a meal, use a divided plate (or your imagination) to help you perfect your portions.

4. Walk at an easy pace for 10-15 minutes.

Nutrition Facts

8 servings per container
Serving size   **2/3 cup (55g)**

Amount per serving
Calories   230

	% Daily Value*
Total Fat 8g	**10%**
Saturated Fat 1g	**5%**
Trans Fat 0g	
Cholesterol 0mg	**0%**
Sodium 160mg	**7%**
Total Carbohydrate 37g	**13%**
Dietary Fiber 4g	**14%**
Total Sugars 12g	
Includes 10g Added Sugars	**20%**
Protein 3g	
Vitamin D 2mcg	10%
Calcium 260mg	20%
Iron 8mg	45%
Potassium 235mg	6%

* The % Daily Value (DV) tells you how much a nutrient in a serving of food contributes to a daily diet. 2,000 calories a day is used for general nutrition advice.

Chapter Nine

Carb Counting the Easy Way

CARB COUNTING IS A great way to keep your blood sugars on a more even keel. When I teach carb counting, my clients are so relieved to know that they can still have their favorite foods without "going off the wagon." They walk out of the office feeling like they've been given a gift — the gift of eating for pleasure again. Using carb counting, you can enjoy good food and good health!

Why use carb counting for diabetes management?

If you've read up on macronutrients, you know that carbohydrates are the only foods that significantly raise your blood sugar. Carb counting is an easier solution than the old

Diabetic Exchange System, which requires you to count up every single portion of food you eat (whether it raises your blood sugar or not). With carb counting, you only need to worry about the foods that will raise your blood glucose, and you can stop stressing about the rest of what you eat.

Which foods count as carbs?

Speaking broadly, anything in these categories of food counts as a carbohydrate:

- Starchy foods like bread, cereal, rice, and pasta
- Fruit and fruit juices
- Milk and yogurt
- Starchy vegetables like potatoes, corn, and peas
- Chips and pretzels
- Cakes, pies, cookies, ice cream, and candy

Don't worry — you can still have carbs even if you want to manage your diabetes!

I know what you might be thinking because I've introduced the concept of carb counting to lots of people with diabetes. When they see this list, most people say, "What! Are you saying I can't have any of those foods????"

That's not what I'm saying. I am saying that you'll have to pay attention to how much and how often you eat those foods.

These are the basics of carb counting for diabetes:

1. At **each meal**, you'll have a recommended amount of carbohydrates. Your personal recommendation depends on your age, gender, and activity level. Generally, the recommendation varies from 30 grams per meal for very petite, older, sedentary women, to 75 grams per meal for very active young men. Forty-five to sixty grams of carbohydrate per meal is a good starting point for the average person.

2. Think of your personal carbohydrate recommendation like a budget. Let's imagine that my personal carb

recommendation is forty-five grams per meal. At each meal, I imagine that $45 suddenly appears in my pocket. I can use the money for that meal but if I don't, it will disappear out of my pocket. I can't decide not to have any carbs for breakfast, add those 45 grams of carbs to my 45 grams at lunch, and then splurge on 90 grams worth of carbohydrate. If I did, my blood sugar would soar. I have to stay within my budget at each meal so that I can keep my blood sugar in check.

3. I can eat anything I want within my budget. Obviously, it would be better for me to spend my carbohydrate "dollars" on high-quality foods like beans than it would for me to eat chocolate bars. And, the more fiber I eat, the smaller spike I'll experience in my blood sugar after a meal. But...it's my "money" and I can do what I want. So, if a dish of beans and rice is worth 45 grams of carbohydrate and so is a candy bar, and I really want a candy bar, that's my decision to make.

Count carbs by the meal, not by the day

Notice that your carbohydrate budget is specific to each meal, not per day. It's not OK to add up all the carbs you get for each meal and snack, lump them all together, and come up with a daily carb limit.

Think about the rise in your blood sugar after you eat carbs as a wave in the ocean. We want short little waves in our blood glucose, not giant tsunami-like swells. Just like the average shoreline, your body can handle short little waves a lot better than it can handle a tsunami. Spacing your carbs out throughout the day results in short little waves of increased blood sugar. If you eat no carbs all day long and then eat all of your carb "budget" at dinner, you're setting yourself up for a blood sugar tsunami.

How to read a food label to count carbs for diabetes

1. Look for "Total Carbohydrate" on the label. Make note of the number of grams of carbohydrate in the food.

2. Find the "Serving Size" at the top of the food label. Now you know how much food

you're dealing with.

3. But...It's important that you know that the Total Carbohydrate on the label refers only to the Serving Size the labels references. In other words, the label won't usually tell you how many grams of carbs there are in the whole container. (I was talking about this with a friend who was drinking a 20 oz. soft drink. She looked at the soft drink and noted that the label said there were 26 grams of carbohydrate. But...the label was only referencing the serving size, 8 oz. The full size of the soft drink was 20 oz., and she didn't understand this at first.)

4. To determine the grams of carbohydrate in the whole container of food, you would need to multiply the Total Carbohydrate by the Servings per Container.

5. Now you know how many grams of carbohydrate are in the serving size shown at the top of the food label, and how many grams of carbohydrate there are in the whole container. In the case of my friend's 20 oz soda, a serving has 26

grams of carb, but the whole container has 66 grams of carb.

6. Decide whether or not you want to "spend" your carbs on this particular food. Do you like yogurt enough to spend 30 grams of carbohydrate on a 4 oz container? If you do, great. If that seems like a waste of carbohydrates to you, you can decide not to spend your carbs on that food. Maybe you'd rather have 2 slices of bread instead of the container of yogurt — it's up to you.

7. The sugars listed on the food label are already included in the Total Carbohydrate. You don't need to focus on them.

8. The more fiber in the food, the more slowly it will be digested, and that's a good thing. Some people like to subtract fiber from carbs to get "net carbs." If you're just starting out with carb counting, there's no need to get fancy. All you need to think about is the Serving Size and the Total Carbohydrate.

Benefits of carb counting for diabetes

Carb counting lets you keep your blood sugar in check and enjoy foods you love. You can eat good nutritious food most of the time, and also realize that a handful of chips or a couple of cookies is not completely off-limits as long as you "budget" for them.

Carb counting gives you the freedom to eat what you like and keep your blood sugar numbers where you want them, too.

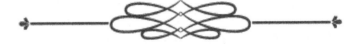

Day 9 Action Items

1. Start reading food labels for carbohydrates by following these steps:

- Look at the label on your favorite carbohydrate food.

- Find the "Total Carbohydrate".

- Find the "Servings per Container".

- Multiply the Total Carbohydrate by the Servings per container.

- Your result is the total number of grams of carbohydrate in the box, can, or bottle.

- Does this food or drink fit in your "budget"?

2. **Walk at an easy pace for 10-15 minutes. Stretch for 2 minutes, then walk at a brisk pace for 5-10 minutes.**

Chapter Ten

Calculate Your Personal Carbohydrate Needs

IF YOU HAVE TYPE 2 diabetes, you've probably wondered how to determine your daily carb requirement. Today, we'll answer that question.

Previously, I wrote about how to accomplish carbohydrate counting, as well as an easier way to manage blood sugars called the Plate Method. Today, I'll walk you through the steps you need to take to determine your personal daily carbohydrate needs. Then, we'll break that down into a specific amount of carb for each meal and snack.

Factors Affecting Your Daily Carb Requirement

Each person is unique, and so is his or her body's daily carb requirement. Your body's need for Calories and carbohydrates varies depending on several factors:

1. Age: As a general rule, the younger you are, the higher your metabolism. A person who needs 2,000 Calories a day at age 20 may only need 1,200 Calories a day at age 70. I know that's not fair, but it's true.

2. Gender: Men usually need more Calories and carbs than women because they carry more muscle mass.

3. Weight and muscle mass: The more muscular you are, the more Calories and carbs you burn at rest.

4. Physical activity level: The more active you are, the more Calories and carbs you'll burn off, and the more Calories and carbs you'll need to eat to maintain your weight.

5. Anti-diabetic medication or insulin dose (if you take either of those): If you tend toward hypoglycemia (low blood sugar) you may have a tendency to "feed the insulin." This happens when people are afraid of going low, so they overeat rather

than using less medication. If you're in this crowd, I don't blame you — low blood sugar feels bad and it's scary, but eating to keep your blood sugar up when you're overmedicated in counter-productive. This is an issue that will need to be worked out with the help of your Certified Diabetes Care and Education Specialist.

Daily Carb Requirement Calculator

Input your information into my calculator to get an estimate of your daily carb requirements. Visit www.juliecunninghamrd.com/resources to find the calculator.

Understanding Your Daily Carb Requirement Calculator Results

You probably noticed that we didn't calculate grams of carb needed per day. Instead, we calculated grams of carb needed per meal and per snack. That's because our bodies need to take in smaller, regular doses of carbohydrates to keep our blood sugar levels on an even keel. We don't want to eat a paltry amount of carbs all day long, and then go crazy "spending" all of our carbs in the evening.

The results you got from the calculator are an estimate of the number of grams of carbohydrate you need at each of 3 meals and 3 snacks per day. If you already count carbs and you have a system that's working for you, then, by all means, stick with what's working. If you take insulin or an anti-diabetic medication that comes with the risk of hypoglycemia (such as sulfonylurea), please consult your healthcare team before changing your carb intake and/or your medications. This calculator is not a substitute for personal medical advice.

Are snacks required as part of my daily carb requirement?

I get lots of questions about whether snacks are required. The answer is no, not usually.

If your blood sugar is low, you already know that you'll have to have to treat that low with simple carbohydrates to bring it up. If you have repeated lows, you probably need to talk with your healthcare team about adjusting your medication.

Most people who ask this question about snacks aren't talking about treating hypoglycemia. They're just asking about everyday eating. If your blood sugar is normal or high and you're not hungry, there's no reason to snack. You'll only end up increasing your blood sugar and gaining weight you probably don't want to gain.

Does my daily carb requirement have any wiggle room?

Now you know approximately how many grams of carbohydrates you need to shoot for at each meal and snack. You can use your label reading and carb counting skills to help you stick to your carbohydrate "budget." It would be almost impossible to get exactly the same number of grams of carbohydrate at every meal, and that's OK. If you stay within 10% of your goal, you're doing great. For example, if your recommended amount of carbohydrate at each meal is 45 grams, but you can stay between 41 and 49 grams at each meal, you're doing beautifully.

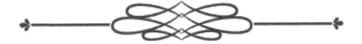

Day 10 Action Items

1. Use the calculator on my resources page to estimate your meal and snack-time carbohydrate needs: https://www.juliecunninghamrd.com/resources

2. Walk at an easy pace for 15-20 minutes. Stretch for 2 minutes.

Chapter Eleven

Meal Plans

MEAL PLANS FOR DIABETES can save you a ton of stress. They can help keep your blood sugar in good control, cut down on your grocery bill, and save you all the time it takes to think about what you want to eat, how much food you need to buy, and what you need to do to get it on the table.

Some people don't like the idea of meal plans because they don't want anyone else to tell them what to eat, and that's OK. If you're that person, you can use the plate method and/or carb counting to help you determine what to eat.

If you prefer an efficient system that combines carb counting with grocery shopping and recipes so you'll always have an answer to the question, "What's for dinner?" then meal planning might be the best choice for you.

Why use a meal plan for diabetes?

You may have heard the quote from Lewis Carroll, "If you don't know where you want to go, any road will take you there." That's true in many situations, including health. If you don't know how you want to change your health, you can eat almost anything and wait to see what happens. But, if you know that you want to improve your health, you've got to stay on the path that will lead you there. A meal plan is an eating plan for better health.

Types of meal plans for diabetes

There are different types of meal plans. Some are very specific — they come with nutrient analysis, cooking instructions, and grocery shopping lists. There are meal plans that are a lot less intense — just a menu.

Options for diabetes-friendly meal plans

1. You're welcome to sign up for my free 5-day diabetes-friendly meal plan at www.juliecunninghamrd.com

2. Living Plate offers a 3-day trial of their diabetes meal plan. After that, this is the least expensive of all Registered Dietitian-created meal planning options. At the time of publication, the fee is $9 per month.* If you'd lie a free trial of living plate, visit this webpage: https://www.livingplaterx.com/juliecunninghamrd/diabetes/signup

3. EatLovePro is the service I use to provide my clients with custom-tailored meal plans. Customized meal plans include 3 meals and a snack every day, plus a grocery shopping list, cooking instructions, and nutrition information. EatLovePro also comes with a smartphone app that my clients can use. If you'd like to access personalized meal planning via EatLovePro, visit my website at juliecunninghamrd.com/meal-planning.

4. Make your own meal plan using a calendar: each day as you make a diabetes-friendly dinner, write it down on your calendar. At the end of the month, you'll have 30 days worth of diabetes-friendly meals recorded. You can keep that page of your calendar and continue to rotate through those same meals. (Most people make the same eight or ten meals over and over again, so you'll be ahead of the pack as far as a variety if you get 30 meals on your calendar).

5. Make your own meal plan using index cards. Similar to the last point, write down each diabetes-friendly dinner you make for 30 days, but instead of using a calendar, use index cards. Put the meal on the front (salmon, salad, roast potatoes...). On the back, list the ingredients you need for the meal (3 pounds salmon, 1 bag baby spinach, 8 oz goat cheese...). Keep your index cards secured together with a rubber band. Each time you need a dinner idea, grab the card on top and take it with you to the grocery store (or to work and then to the store). You'll never have to wonder what to make or forget to buy

something essential. After you make that meal, the card goes to the back of the stack, and you won't see it again for another 30 meals, so you won't get bored of eating the same thing over and over again.

Do I have to use a diabetes meal plan to keep my blood sugar in good control?

No. You don't have to do anything you don't want to do! You might be one of those people who is very successful using the plate method or counting carbs in your head, and that's just fine. Meal planning makes life easier for some people, and it annoys other people. So decide what makes your life easier and do that. Meal planning is just one more tool that might help you get your blood sugar where you want it. You get to decide what works for you!

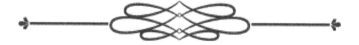

Day 11 Action Items

1. Decide whether or not you'd like to give meal plans for diabetes a try.

2. If so, take a look at the meal planning methods above and choose one to try this week.

3. Walk at an easy pace for 10-15 minutes, stretch for 2 minutes, and then walk at a brisk pace for 5-10 minutes.

Carb Content of
Alcoholic Drinks

Information provided is for the serving size specified only and does not include any mixers additives that may be consumed with alcohol. Information taken from USDA data.

	SERVING SIZE	CARBS	CALORIES	GRAMS ALCOHOL
BEER	12 oz	13 grams	153	14
LIGHT BEER	12 oz	5-9 grams	105	11
"ULTRA" BEER	12 oz	1-3 grams	95	10
WHITE WINE	5 oz	4 grams	125	15
RED WINE	5 oz	4 grams	122	16
80 PROOF SPIRITS	1.5 oz	0 grams	97	14

Chapter Twelve

Alcohol and Diabetes

FIRST, BEFORE I WRITE this post about diabetes and alcohol, I have to say that I'm almost a teetotaler, and I don't want to encourage anyone who doesn't drink to start. There is almost no benefit to drinking alcohol and there are plenty of risks. Having said that, I know that lots of people drink alcohol and don't plan to stop. They need help figuring out how to navigate drinking alcohol without getting their blood sugars out of whack. So, here goes...

If you think diabetes and alcohol can't mix, you might like what you're about to read. Many of my clients are surprised to learn that they can still enjoy some of their favorite adult beverages while keeping their blood sugars in good control. But don't break open the bottle just yet — there are some caveats that come with imbibing when you have diabetes, and you'll need to know what to watch out for.

Alcohol may lower blood sugar

Alcohol prevents the liver from releasing sugar into the bloodstream, so a person with diabetes who drinks pure alcohol would see a drop in their blood sugar levels.

But…some alcoholic beverages, like beer, naturally contain carbohydrates. While the alcohol in the beer lowers blood sugar, the carbs in the beer raise blood sugar. Most of the time, the carbs win this battle and the overall effect of drinking a regular beer is a rise in your blood sugar. But each person is different, so you'll need to check your blood sugar more often if and when you drink.

Carbohydrate content of alcoholic drinks

As you can see on the chart, spirits such as vodka and rum have little to no carbohydrates. If you drink them straight or with a sugar-free mixer like a diet soda or sparkling water, your blood sugar is likely to go down.

The "mixers" are usually the problem when blood sugar spikes after drinking alcohol. Regular sodas, juices, and flavorings like grenadine are very high in carbs. These add-ons are really the culprit when blood sugar spikes after drinking liquor. Think rum-and-Coke, vodka-and-OJ, or Pina Coladas.

Diabetes, alcohol, and your long-term health

I'm sure you don't need me to tell you that drinking too much alcohol can lead to a host of serious problems, like these:

- High blood pressure, heart disease, and stroke
- Liver disease
- Cancer of the breast, mouth, throat, esophagus, liver, and colon

- A weakened immune system, increasing your chances of getting sick

- Memory problems, like dementia

- Depression and anxiety

- Alcohol dependence/addiction

The recommendation is that women drink no more than one alcoholic beverage each day and that men limit their intake of alcoholic beverages to two per day. And no...you can't save them all up and have them on Friday night! (I've been asked that question at least a thousand times.)

How to mix diabetes and alcohol

If you have diabetes, drinking alcohol requires a little more attention than it would if you didn't have diabetes. (No surprise there!) Here's what you need to do to stay safe:

- Check your blood sugar before you drink alcohol

- Know how many grams of carbs are in your alcoholic beverages

- If you use meal-time insulin, bolus for the carbs in the alcohol just like you would

for carbs in food

•   Check your blood sugar again 1-2 hours after drinking alcohol. If you continue to drink (which I have to say again is not recommended), continue to check your blood sugar every 1-2 hours.

•   Be prepared and have supplies ready in case of high blood sugar or low blood sugar emergencies.

Diabetes and alcohol can mix, as long as you consider the carbs in the alcohol and the fact that the alcohol itself will likely decrease your blood sugar. Pay attention to how your body reacts to alcohol — because everybody is different. If you have diabetes, you can have an alcoholic drink every now and then. Like everyone else, you just need to know your own limits.

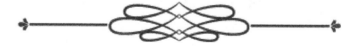

Day 12 Action Items

1. If you don't drink alcohol, great. Skip to #8 below.

2. If you drink alcohol, use the Carb Content of Alcoholic Drinks chart to learn how many grams of carbohydrate are in one standard drink of your favorite beverage.

3. Think about whether you normally drink a "standard" size beverage, or whether your normal drink is smaller or larger than the size on the chart. Measure it out if you need to.

4. Do the math to determine how many grams of carbs you normally drink in your alcohol alone (grams of carb in a standard serving x number of standard servings you consume).

5. Repeat the same process with any mixers you use.

6. Is it worth it, or are you blowing your carbohydrate budget beverages before you even get to those bar snacks?

7. Could you switch to a light or an ultralight beer or a sugar-free mixer? If

you did, how much would that change your carbohydrate intake?

8. Walk at an easy pace for 15-20 minutes, then stretch for 2 minutes.

Chapter Thirteen

Sugars vs. Alternative Sweeteners

I HAVE CLIENTS WITH diabetes who worry that using sweeteners will cause them to have other health problems in the future. They've heard rumors that sweeteners are related to weight gain or even cancer. I don't blame them a bit for wanting to be cautious, but I do want to help them (and you) make an informed decision about whether to use sugar or an alternative sweetener if you have diabetes.

The truth is, alternative and artificial sweeteners can add a whole lot of enjoyment to an eating plan that might not otherwise be so sweet. If you have diabetes, it's perfectly

OK to use alternative sweeteners to add a little sweetness to your diet and your life.

Sweeteners used as sugar alternatives

Each of these sweeteners has very few or no calories and can be used to replace sugar:

- Aspartame

- Acesulfame K

- Advantame

- Monk Fruit

- Neotame

- Saccharine

- Stevia

- Sucralose

What research says about alternative sweeteners

What if I told you that eating margarine is associated with getting a divorce in Maine? Would you believe that eating margarine causes divorce? No...that would be silly. It's true that between the years 2000-2009, margarine consumption and divorce rates in the state of Maine were correlated by more than 99%, but that doesn't mean that one caused the other.

Research tells us that people who regularly use alternative sweeteners are heavier than people who don't. Sometimes, people who hear this draw the conclusion that sweeteners cause weight gain. That's not necessarily true. Just like with margarine and Maine divorces, sweetener consumption is associated with higher weight, but that doesn't mean sweetener consumption is the cause of higher weight. It could be that people who are already heavier tend to choose alternative sweeteners because they are trying to manage their weight.

Believing that sweeteners cause weight gain is like believing that margarine causes divorce. We just don't have any good solid proof of that.

Do sugar-sweetened drinks cause health problems?

A high intake of sweetened drinks is associated with heart disease, but they may not be the cause of that heart disease. People who drink sugary beverages are more likely to have other not-so-healthy habits, like smoking or choosing not to exercise. Just because sugary drinks are associated with heart disease doesn't mean that sugary drinks cause heart disease.

What we know for sure is that sugar is a form of carbohydrate and that all carbohydrates, especially simple carbs like sugar, will raise your blood sugar. If you have diabetes, you probably don't want to raise your blood sugar unless you're experiencing hypoglycemia (low blood sugar.) So...**alternative sweeteners are the best choice for most people with type 2 diabetes.**

Is it safe to use artificial sweeteners for a long time?

Some people worry that artificial sweeteners are going to cause them problems down the road. At this time, we don't have any evidence to say that artificially sweetened drinks are associated with health problems like heart disease or cancer.

We do know that the consumption of artificial sweeteners is associated with higher weight. So, we can only make the best choice that we can make today. For me, as a person without diabetes, that comes down to drinking my tea completely unsweetened and my coffee with a little sugar. Let's face it, I'm addicted to my morning caffeine, but I really don't like the taste of black coffee.

If I did have diabetes, I'd choose stevia because it is found in nature. Several other alternative sweeteners such as sucralose, aspartame, & saccharine are man-made. That doesn't make them necessarily bad (cocaine is found in nature too), but it would make me choose stevia instead.

Choosing sweetener vs. sugar if you have diabetes

If you have diabetes, we know that sugar raises your blood sugar right away. The only time we want to see a spike in your blood sugar is if you are experiencing a low. So, the only time that's a good time to have a high-sugar food or drink is when you're trying to treat a low blood sugar. Even then, the recommended amount is 15 grams of carbohydrate or about 4 ounces of juice or real soda.

Since routine consumption of regular sugar is out, people with diabetes who want something sweet should definitely go with the artificially sweetened version. I'm not endorsing the idea of drinking diet soda all day long...I'm just saying that diet soda is the lesser of two evils if you are a person with diabetes, and most people want some "pleasure foods" in their life.

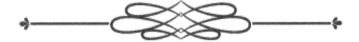

Day 13 Action Items

1. If you're regularly using real sugar (including white, brown, raw, or turbinado sugar), consider using an alternative sweetener. Go back up to the list of alternatives at the top of this article and choose the one you'd like to try.

2. Walk at an easy pace for 15-20 minutes.

Chapter Fourteen

When to Check Your Blood Sugar

KNOWING WHEN TO CHECK blood sugar is important when you have diabetes. You don't want to check unnecessarily, causing yourself pain and wasting your supplies. But you also don't want to avoid checking when you need to check — you might end up with a high or low blood sugar level that you could have treated sooner.

How often do I need to check my blood sugar?

How often you need to check your blood sugar depends on a few factors:

- Do you take insulin?

- Is hypoglycemia unawareness a concern for you?

- Do you take anti-diabetic medications with the potential side effect of hypoglycemia (low blood sugar), such as sulfonylureas?

- Is your blood sugar in good control, or are you trying to work on your A1c right now?

How to decide when to check your blood sugar

For people who take insulin, the plan is pretty simple:

- Blood sugar needs to be tested before any insulin injection

- Test your blood sugar any time you feel unwell

For people with diabetes who don't take insulin, the rules vary a little more:

- If you take no medication or only medications with a low risk of hypoglycemia, you may need to check your blood sugar much less frequently than a person who takes insulin. It's possible that you only need to check a couple of times a week, but always follow the advice of your medical team.

• Always check your blood sugar any time you feel unwell, including when you have any of these symptoms: headache, blurry vision, excessive thirst or urination, sweating, shaking, feeling dizzy, weak, or nervous.

Don't fool yourself when you check your blood sugar

Checking your sugar when you know it'll be low is kind of like when I weigh myself first thing in the morning with no clothes on. I want to get the lowest possible number on the scale. It's a number I couldn't possibly get for the rest of the day. I know I'm going to weigh more than that when I get to my doctor's office, but sometimes I still do it, and I'm only fooling myself.

Randomly checking your blood sugar without any rhyme or reason doesn't give you much information. Waiting until you've "been good" and eaten something low carb so you can check your blood sugar and write down a nice low number in your logbook doesn't really help you either. It's a waste of a finger stick. The truth is going to come out when your A1c is measured, so you might as well be honest with yourself all along.

Use paired testing to check blood sugar

Paired testing is just what it sounds like, testing blood sugar in pairs of two fingersticks. Two blood sugar levels are checked before and after an event, such as a meal or a workout. That way, you can determine how the food you ate or the exercise you did changed your blood sugar levels.

A plan for paired testing

For most people, blood sugar levels peak between one and two hours after a meal. Lots of people check only their fasting (first thing in the morning) blood sugars, and when they get their A1c results, they're unpleasantly surprised. That's because fasting blood sugar can be completely normal even when post-meal blood sugars are out of whack. If you only check fasting blood sugars, you can't possibly know what's going on with your blood sugar levels after your meals.

If you haven't been checking your blood sugar levels and you want to get back into the swing of things, you can use paired testing to play detective.

To implement paired testing, decide which meal of the day you want to work on. Maybe this week it's breakfast. Check your blood sugar just before breakfast, eat your breakfast, and then check your blood sugar again between one and two hours after eating. Write down your blood sugar levels in your logbook, along with your best estimate of how many grams of carbohydrate you ate at breakfast. Do this every day for a week.

Do you notice any patterns? Is one of your usual breakfast meals better than others at keeping your blood sugar levels in the normal range? What can you determine about the way your body is handling the foods you eat?

If your blood sugar stays in range after your meals, that's great. Your detective work is done. If not, there are only three factors you can manipulate to change the outcome — your carbohydrate intake, your activity level, and your medication. If your blood sugars are out of range, talk with your Certified Diabetes Care and Education Specialist about your next step.

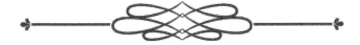

Day 14 Action Items

1. Decide whether paired testing is something you'd like to try. If it is, decide which meal you want to work on this week.

2. If you already have a logbook, great. If not, obtain a small notebook to record your paired testing blood sugar levels.

3. No walking today! — There is rest for the weary, after all.

Chapter Fifteen

What to Do When You Have High Blood Sugar

I SPENT MY HONEYMOON trying to determine how to lower high blood sugar. Not mine — my grandmother's. (This was before I became a diabetes educator, in case you're wondering.) A cousin came to the wedding with a stomach bug and delivered an unwanted "gift" to lots of wedding attendees, including my grandmother and the groom. The honeymoon didn't happen, but we did make a few trips to urgent care.

My grandmother had been diabetic for as long as I could remember, but she made the six-hour trip to my wedding without her glucometer or her diabetes medications. She became miserably sick and dehydrated from the stomach virus. I went to the pharmacy and purchased a glucometer to check her blood sugar, which was off the charts. She refused to go to the ER, so we went to urgent care instead. I don't remember how high her blood glucose was, but I remember that the urgent care doc wanted her to go to the ER. She declined. We were sent home with enough diabetic medication to last her until she returned to her house, and I was worried about her safety.

What makes blood sugar spike when you usually have good control?

My grandma's blood sugar was elevated because she had a fever, an infection (the stomach bug) and because she was dehydrated. People react differently to all kinds of stressors, but these are the things that generally cause high blood sugar in a person whose diabetes is normally in good control:

- Fever
- Infection
- Dehydration

- Stress

- High carbohydrate intake

- Skipping diabetes medication or insulin

- Taking steroid medications

Signs and symptoms of high blood sugar

You may feel one, some, or all of these things if your blood sugar is high — then again, there are some people who don't feel anything:

- Headache

- Extreme thirst

- Extreme hunger

- Excessive urination

- Blurry vision

- Weight loss, in more severe and long-term cases

- Long-term: recurring infection & cuts that won't heal

What blood sugar level is considered too high?

- If you have diabetes, the American Diabetes Association recommends that your post-meal blood sugar stays under 180.

- If your blood glucose reaches 250 mg/dL, take steps to bring it down.

- A blood glucose level of 300 mg/dL may require medical attention.

How to lower a high blood sugar level

You may be able to lower your blood sugar level at home by taking the steps below. If you try these steps and you're not successful, seek the advice of a physician.

1. Drink 2-3 large glasses of water. This will combat dehydration. (Don't drink sugary beverages, including sports drinks such as Gatorade or Powerade.)

2. Take a walk. Walking for 30 minutes or more may help bring your blood sugar down. (Don't exercise strenuously.)

3. Rest or meditate. If stress is causing your blood sugar to increase, rest or meditation may help to lower your blood sugar.

4. Continue to take your diabetes medications or insulin as prescribed by your physician.

5. If you try the steps above and you see no improvement (or a worsening) of your blood sugar levels, call your physician for advice.

A lot of times, clients tell me that they feel guilty when their blood glucose levels are high. If you look at the list of causes above, you can see that there are lots of reasons why your blood glucose level might be high that don't have anything to do with whether or not you eat "perfectly." Besides, nobody's perfect. So, give yourself a break. If your blood sugar level is too high, take the steps you need to take to address it. If you can't get it down on your own, call your doctor — their job is to help you figure out your next steps when you've already done what you can do on your own, and they want to help.

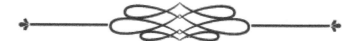

Day 15 Action Items

1. Think about your usual blood sugar levels. Everyone is different. Where is your "cut-off point?" At what level do you need to take steps to lower your blood glucose? At what blood glucose level do you need to call your physician?

2. Write those two numbers down: the level at which you'll try to lower your blood sugar and the level at which you'll need to call your doctor.

3. Write down the number for your physician, the nearest urgent care, and 911. Post the numbers in a convenient location or program them into your smartphone. (I know you already know the number "911", but you'd be surprised how many people can't remember that number in a true emergency.)

4. Good! You're all set, just in case you have a high blood glucose emergency.

5. Walk at an easy pace for 10-15 minutes, then a brisk pace for 5-10 minutes. Finish with a 2-minute stretch.

Low blood sugar treatment

Blood Glucose Level

	LESS THAN 55	56-70	ABOVE 70
JUICE	8 ounces	4 ounces	Not required
REAL SODA (NOT DIET)	10 ounces	5 ounces	Not required
GLUCOSE TABS	6 tabs	3 tabs	Not required
HARD CANDY (NOT SUGAR-FREE)	10 pieces	5 pieces	Not required

After you decide what to use to treat your blood sugar, wait 15-20 minutes and check your blood sugar level again.   If your blood glucose if above 70, have a meal or a snack. If not, repeat treatment every 20 minnutes or call your doctor or 911 if you're unable to improve your blood sugar.

Each serving of food under the <55 mg/dL column provides approximately 30 grams CHO, and each serving under the 56-70 mg/dL column provides approximately 15 grams CHO.

Chapter Sixteen

How to Manage Low Blood Sugar

YEARS AGO, I WORKED in cardiac rehab. One of our patients had diabetes, and he had an episode of low blood sugar during his workout. He started slurring his words, sweating and stumbling around like a drunk person. I checked his blood sugar and saw that it was down in the 40s. We gave him two of the juice boxes that we kept stored just for that purpose, and we waited for a nerve-wracking 20 minutes for his blood sugar to come up. Finally, it did. Our patient felt a little tired but generally OK. He ate some peanut butter crackers, skipped the rest of his workout, and went home.

I've never worked on the inpatient side of a hospital if I could help it — I don't do blood or guts or gore very well. Acute healthcare isn't interesting to me; it's scary. I was scared for my patient that day, and I've been scared for other patients since that day too. That's why I want you to be prepared to handle a low blood sugar emergency if you need to.

Who's at risk for hypoglycemia (low blood sugar)?

- People who take insulin
- Those who take anti-diabetic medications with the risk of hypoglycemia, such as sulfonylureas
- People who take diabetes medications and skip meals
- Those who exercise without checking their blood sugar first

What blood sugar numbers are considered low?

- A blood sugar level of less than 70 mg/dL is considered hypoglycemia.
- A blood sugar level of less than 55 mg/dL is considered severe hypoglycemia.

How do I treat low blood glucose?

You've already read the information on macronutrients and diabetes, and you know that the only foods that raise your blood sugar are carbohydrates. Ordinarily, you'll want to limit your carbs to keep your blood glucose from rising too high. But when your blood sugar is low, you need carbs to help you increase your blood sugar.

When blood sugar is low, you want to get it up to normal as quickly as possible. That means eating or drinking simple carbohydrates that can be easily digested and absorbed by your body, not carbs that come with added fiber to slow your gut down.

Try not to overcompensate when your sugar is low

If you've ever had a low, you know how bad it feels. Most people with hypoglycemia want to eat anything and everything they can find to get their blood sugar up right that minute. I don't blame them, but that just doesn't work. If you eat fat and protein along with your simple carbohydrates, you'll actually slow down your digestion, delaying the time it takes for your blood sugar to come up to normal. You're really prolonging your agony if you have a low and you eat anything but simple carbs.

It takes 15-20 minutes for the sugar to get into your gut, get processed, and hit your bloodstream. The only way to speed that up is to take a glucagon shot or to get IV glucose administered in a hospital or a clinic. If you're feeling bad but still able to function, the best thing to do is choose juice, soda, glucose tabs, or hard candy and eat them quickly. Then wait twenty minutes and check your blood sugar again.

Do I need a glucagon pen?

If you've had repeated episodes of hypoglycemia, especially severe lows, or if you have needed EMS to help you due to a low blood sugar attack, a glucagon pen may be right for you.

What is a glucagon pen?

Glucagon is a hormone that naturally occurs in the body. Think of it as the opposite hormone from insulin. Instead of lowering blood sugar, glucagon raises blood sugar. If you're at risk for hypoglycemia, your healthcare provider can write a prescription for you to have a glucagon pen.

It's important that you know how to use your glucagon pen if you have one, but it's even more important that your friends, family, and coworkers know how to use it. They also need to know where you keep your glucagon pen. (It needs to stay with you all the time — keeping it in your kitchen won't do you much good if your blood sugar runs low at work.)

Be prepared for a hypoglycemic emergency

Hopefully, you never have a hypoglycemic emergency, but better to be safe than sorry. In the action steps below, you'll get prepared to handle a low.

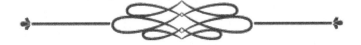

Day 16 Action Items

1. Make copies of the low blood sugar treatment chart if you'd like. You might like a copy at home, in the car, at work, etc.

2. Decide whether you'd like to treat your lows with juice, soda, hard candy, or glucose tabs. (There are other things you can use, but we'll stick with those for now.) If you choose to treat with juice, kid-size juice boxes are especially good. They're the right size and they don't need refrigeration.

3. Purchase or gather the foods/beverages you've decided to use for treatment.

4. Think of all the places you might need to treat and store enough to treat one severe low or two moderately low blood sugar levels at each of these places:

- Bedside table
- Beside your chair in the living room or den

- Kitchen (Label your soda or juice as "do not drink" so your family won't accidentally use it.)

- Car

- Office

5. Walk at an easy pace for 10-15 minutes and then walk at a brisk pace for 5-10 minutes. Stretch for 2 minutes.

Chapter Seventeen

Continuous Glucose Monitors

WONDERING IF YOU CAN use a continuous glucose monitor for type 2 diabetes? Yes, you can, and I love these little devices!

A few years ago, I worked in the wellness division of a hospital. It was my team's job to screen over 12,000 employees for their cholesterol and blood sugar levels. This required getting what seemed like a half-pint of blood out of a finger stick, and we used pretty big lancets to do the job.

I stuck my own finger for the test, and I really hit a nerve! This sounds whiny — and wimpy — but I'm not kidding when I say that I had little twinges of pain in that finger off and on for six weeks.

I can only imagine how torturous it must be for those of you who have to stick yourselves multiple times a day, every day. Truly, I feel for you. This brings me to why I love continuous glucose monitors, also known as CGMs. They allow the wearer to avoid almost all fingersticks!

How do continuous glucose monitors work?

CGMs consists of three main components:

- Sensors
- Transmitters
- Readers (receivers)

CGM sensors

With CGMs, a very thin wire is inserted just under your skin. The wire stays there for 10-14 days, depending on the brand of the device. This wire is called a sensor because it "senses" the amount of sugar in your bloodstream. The sensor is secured to your body with medical-grade tape.

CGM transmitters and receivers

A transmitter is then attached to the sensor. The transmitter is the technology that takes the information from the sensor and communicates it to the reader where you can see your blood sugar levels. You can also read your blood sugar levels on your smartphone after downloading an app.

A continuous glucose monitor can help you lower your A1c

Of course, there's the benefit of eliminating finger sticks. But people who use CGMs are able to lower their A1cs because they get lots of information about how their bodies react to different foods and insulin doses. They also get information not just about where their blood sugar levels are right now, but where their blood sugar levels are headed. That makes a huge difference in their diabetes management. For example, if you know that your blood sugar is rapidly falling, you can eat something before you're low, saving yourself from the miserable feeling of hypoglycemia and the time it takes to recover from that misery.

CGMs available in the US today

There are two main brands of CGMs available to people with diabetes in the US today:

• Freestyle Libre is wearable for 14 days. It does not require fingerstick calibration. The Libre does require that the user wave the reader over the sensor in order to get a blood glucose measurement. The Freestyle Libre does **not** come with built-in alarms to let you know if you're running too high or too low.

• Dexcom is wearable for 10 days, and it also does not require fingerstick calibration. Dexcom checks your blood sugar every five minutes with no action required on your part, and it comes with a built-in alarm to let you know if your blood sugars are outside the range you set.

Medtronic and Senseonic also make continuous glucose monitors, but at this time, they both require two fingersticks a day, so I don't recommend them.

The cost of continuous glucose monitors

Your insurance company may cover the cost of a CGM. These are the approximate cash prices for the devices:

- Freestyle: A one-time cost of $70-$100 for the reader, and about $125 a month for the sensors.

- Dexcom: Costco offers Dexcom discounts for members. At this time, advertised fees are a one-time cost of $218 for the receiver, $318 for a 3-pack of sensors, and $146 for a transmitter, bringing the monthly cost after the purchase of the receiver to approximately $450. Clearly, Dexcom is the more expensive option.

Who is a candidate for a CGM?

Medicare requires that a person meet these criteria before they will pay for a CGM:

1. Have a diagnosis of diabetes, either type 1 or type 2

2. Routinely monitor blood sugar at home at least four times a day

3. Use 3 or more insulin injections per day OR be on an insulin pump

4. Need frequent insulin adjustments based on blood sugar readings

Other insurance companies may have different criteria, but typically insurance companies follow the same criteria as Medicare when it comes to allowing costs. If you want your insurance company to cover a CGM, you'll need to check your policy to see if they have any particular requirements other than a doctor's prescription.

Which continuous glucose monitor is best for me?

I strongly prefer the Dexcom because it continuously checks your blood sugar without you thinking about it and because it will alert you to highs and lows. If you're asleep and your blood sugar dips down to a dangerously low 55, Dexcom will alarm to wake you up, and Freestyle won't. I think that's critically important.

Having said that, any CGM is better than no CGM, so if your insurance company will only cover the Freestyle, then, by all means, take it!

The bottom line about continuous glucose monitors

•   If finger sticks don't bother you but technology does, CGMs are not a good fit for you.

•   If you'd love to stop sticking your fingers and your insurance will cover it, consider a CGM.

•   If you're afraid to go to bed at night because you're not sure if your blood sugar will bottom out while you're sleeping, Dexcom may help you get a good night's rest.

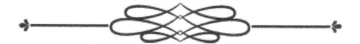

Day 17 Action Items

1. If you avoid checking your blood sugar because you dislike finger sticks — and who could blame you — find out whether or not you're a candidate for a CGM.

2. Use the criteria above if you are covered by Medicare.

3. If you have private insurance, call your insurance company and ask whether they cover CGMs, what criteria you need to meet, and if they have a preferred device.

4. Walk at a brisk pace for 20-25 minutes.

NON-INSULIN MEDICATION FOR TYPE 2 DIABETES

JULIE CUNNINGHAM

NUTRITION

juliecunninghamrd.com

	Risk of hypoglycemia	Weight change	Cost	Pill or Injection
Metformin	NO	NONE/MILD LOSS	LOW	PILL
SGLT2 Inhibitors	NO	LOSS	HIGH	PILL
GLP-1 RA's	NO	LOSS	HIGH	INJECTION
DPP 4 Inhibitors	NO	NO EFFECT	HIGH	PILL
TZDs	NO	GAIN	LOW	PILL
Sulfonylureas	YES	GAIN	LOW	PILL

Chapter Eighteen

Non-Insulin Medications

ALMOST EVERY DAY, A client tells me, "I'll do anything to keep from taking medications for type 2 diabetes." Sometimes clients say, "I know I'm a failure at losing weight and watching what I eat, and that's why I have to take this medicine."

I get it. I don't like taking pills either, but I take medication to prevent migraines every day. Then again, I thank God for the really smart people who figured out which medications would prevent me from having migraines. If I didn't have those medications, I would spend a lot of time in pain, not to mention experiencing the nausea that comes with migraines.

You might be thinking, "Well, that's fine for you...but migraines are different than diabetes." That's true, but did you know that in ancient times migraine sufferers were believed to be possessed by evil spirits? They routinely had their skulls cut open to let the evil spirits out!

Today, people who suffer from type 2 diabetes are frequently blamed for their conditions, too. Sometimes, even healthcare providers blame people with type 2 diabetes for having poor self-control around food or for being "too lazy" to exercise.

The truth is, we're living in a world that almost begs us to sit still and overeat. Unless we have physical jobs (which are fewer and fewer these days), we have to actively work to get exercise. Our options for cheap, high-calorie foods are almost limitless, and that's not helping either. I'm not saying you shouldn't eat well and exercise; you should. I'm also saying that everyone deserves a little grace, and it's not my job to judge you if you're snacking on something other than seaweed.

When is it OK to use medication for type 2 diabetes?

If your A1c is above 7, it may be appropriate to use medication. It's also appropriate to work on your diet and exercise while you use the medication.

Recognize that if you are resistant to taking a medication that your doctor recommends, you may be getting microvascular damage to your eyes, nerves, and kidneys while you "wait and see" if you can get your blood sugar to come down. I'm all for improving your diet and increasing your exercise, and I'm all for controlling your blood sugars as best you can while you make improvements.

Medications for type 2 diabetes

Here's a list of the different classes of medications for type 2 diabetes. Each class of medications may be sold under different brand names.

1. **Metformin**: the first medication for type 2 diabetes. Metformin is very often the first medication that a person with type 2

diabetes or prediabetes is prescribed. Metformin decreases the amount of glucose (sugar) produced by your liver and helps your body's cells use the insulin you produce more efficiently.

2. **Sulfonylureas** work by increasing the amount of insulin produced by the pancreas. I think of them as "pancreas squeezers." These work better in the early stages of type 2 diabetes when a person still has beta-cell function. Sulfonylureas can cause low blood sugar and are not as frequently recommended now that we have newer medications for diabetes.. Glyburide, glimepiride, and glipizide are common sulfonylureas.

3. **Meglitinides** are more commonly known as Starlix and Prandin. These medications are also "pancreas squeezers." They work much more quickly than the sulfonylureas mentioned above and are meant to be taken no more than 30 minutes before the start of a meal. (Taking them earlier can cause a person to have low blood sugar.)

4. **Thiazolidinediones**: Actos and Avandia can help make your cells less resistant to

the insulin your body produces. These medications have been linked to heart disease and weight gain, so most physicians don't prescribe these medications without trying alternatives first.

5. **DPP-4 Inhibitors**: Januvia, Tradjenta, and Onglyza reduce blood sugars, but they don't have a dramatic effect. They may work best for people without extremely high blood glucose levels.

6. **SGLT2 Inhibitors**: Jardiance, Invokana, and Farxiga are examples of SGLT2 Inhibitors. These medications encourage the kidneys to excrete sugar in the urine. SGLT2 Inhibitors may reduce your risk of heart attack and stroke if you are at high risk for those health conditions. They may also increase your risk of urinary tract infection, yeast infection, diabetic ketoacidosis, and low blood pressure.

7. **GLP-1 Receptor Agonists**: These injectable medications include Byetta, Victoza, and Ozempic. These medications cause the stomach to empty more slowly, which results in lowered blood sugars.

GLP-1 Receptor Agonists are also associated with weight loss. Some people experience nausea with these medications, and there is also an increased risk of pancreatitis.

8. **Insulin.** Insulin comes in a number of types, including regular, NPH, short-acting, and long-acting. Most people with type 2 diabetes don't need insulin until 10-15 years after diagnosis, and some people never need insulin at all.

Each medication for type 2 diabetes has a different action time (the length of time from when you swallow or inject it until it starts to work) as well as different potential side effects. Your doctor will take your personal health history into account when choosing your diabetes medication. Keep in mind that your heart, liver, and kidney function have to be considered when your doctor prescribes a medication for your diabetes.

This chart to the left may help you to talk with your healthcare provider about diabetes medications.

Changing your view about medication for diabetes

Whether you use no medications or several medications to manage your type 2 diabetes, the most important thing to know is that you're "allowed" to do anything you need to do to prevent complications of diabetes. If you need to change your diet and start walking, do it. If you're doing all you can do with your diet (whether or not you're doing what you "should" be doing) and your blood sugar is still too high, it's perfectly OK to use medication to get that sugar under control. Don't beat yourself up, just do what you need to do to prevent long-term complications of diabetes. That's the name of the game.

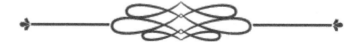

Day 18 Action Items

1. Take a look at the chart. Determine what class of medication you use, if any. Do you have any questions for your

Certified Diabetes Care and Education Specialist, your pharmacist, or your healthcare provider? If so, write your questions down and give your healthcare provider a call.

1. Walk at an easy pace for 10-15 minutes, then walk at a brisk pace for 10-15 minutes. Stretch for 2 minutes.

Normal Metabolism (No Diabetes)

Insulin is the key to helping the body use the carbs/sugar we eat.

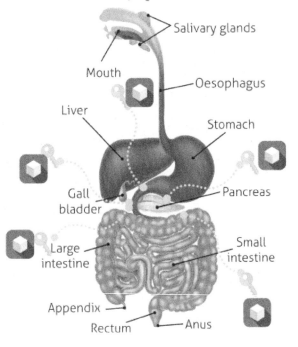

Type 2 Diabetes

Plenty of Insulin, but the key doesn't fit.
The locks on the cells are rusty.

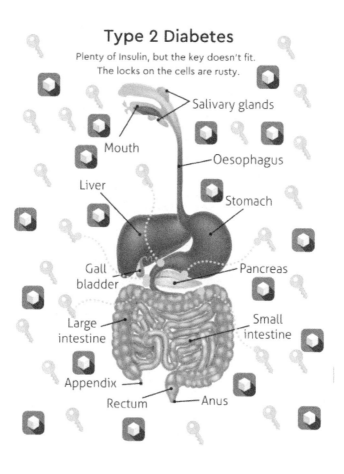

Salivary glands

Mouth

Oesophagus

Liver

Stomach

Gall bladder

Pancreas

Large intestine

Small intestine

Appendix

Rectum

Anus

Chapter Nineteen

Insulin

THE MAIN FUNCTION OF insulin is to help glucose (sugar) move from the bloodstream into the cells. Normally, your pancreas releases insulin when it senses that the level of sugar in the bloodstream is rising. Insulin then "pairs up" with the sugar and helps it cross the border from the bloodstream to the inside of the cells.

I like to think of insulin as a key that fits a lock on the outside of the cells. The key opens the lock on the door to let the sugar inside.

The first picture before this chapter might help you understand the function of insulin in a person without diabetes. Notice that each sugar molecule (cube) is paired up with an insulin molecule (key).

Insulin resistance in type 2 diabetes

If you have type 2 diabetes, you most likely have insulin resistance. This means that your cells won't let insulin do its job — they won't let insulin open the lock and let sugar cross the border to the inside of the cells. I like to think of the locks on the cells of an insulin-resistant person as "rusty." When your cells become insulin resistant, your pancreas starts making lots and lots of insulin. If a pancreas could hope, it would be hoping that one of the keys it makes will fit in the rusty lock (and sometimes that happens, but not often enough).

In the second picture, you see an illustration of the function of insulin in a person with type 2 diabetes. Notice that there is a lot more insulin floating around, and there is also a lot more sugar floating around. Insulin and sugar aren't getting across the border together because of those "rusty locks" on the cells.

The bottom line about the function of insulin

• Insulin is a hormone that helps sugar get into your cells. Cells need sugar because they use it for energy.

• When everything is working correctly, any extra sugar or carbohydrate we eat is stored as fat, in case we need it later.

• Most people with type 2 diabetes have plenty of insulin, but their cells are resistant to it.

Fear of Insulin

Since we've reviewed the function of insulin in type 2 diabetes, let's talk about the fear of insulin. So many people are afraid of insulin, and they usually fall into one of these categories:

• People who are afraid of needles

• Those who are afraid that insulin will make them fat

• People who are afraid that they will take too much insulin and not wake up

• Those who worry that taking insulin means they have failed at taking care of diabetes

So, let's address these fears about insulin one by one:

1. Fear of Insulin Needles

If you're afraid of needles, I hear you. When I was 5, my parents lied to me about going for kindergarten shots because they knew what a giant fit I would pitch. I remember pitching it, too. When the nurse was finished, she tried to give me a coupon for McDonald's french fries, and I said, "I don't want your french fries!" I was generally a sweet, well-behaved kid, but not when it came to shots. My mom still talks about how embarrassed she was that day.

When I became a diabetes educator, I had no experience with injections, other than getting those vaccines as a child. I had to learn to teach people to inject insulin. The best way to do that was to inject myself with saline (which has no effect on blood sugar or anything else).

The first time I did it, I felt mildly nauseous and sweaty. I really, really, really didn't want to stick that needle in my skin. I let the needle hover over my abdomen for a long time before I finally took the plunge. When I finally injected myself, I felt...nothing. As it turns out, insulin needles are so thin, most people don't feel a thing when they inject themselves. So, if you're needle-phobic like me, relax. I promise, if you do need insulin, it's not as bad as you think.

2. **Fear of Fat**

If you think one of the functions of insulin is to make you fat, you're right...sort of. Insulin's job is to help your body store sugar as fuel. If you haven't had enough insulin on board for a while, your sugar (glucose) has been leaving your body without being stored. It's been literally going right down the drain in your urine. So, when you do get enough insulin in your body, and it matches up with the amount of glucose in your bloodstream, some of that glucose gets stored as fat instead of getting lost in the urine. That's normal, and it may also result in weight gain.

3. **Fear of low blood sugar**

Fear of insulin overdose is a legitimate concern. To combat this fear, work with your healthcare team to start small and work up to the insulin dose that's right for you. You don't have to get perfect blood sugars today; you just need to be making progress. Frequent blood sugar checks will also help you to determine whether your insulin dose is appropriate. Lastly, know how to manage low blood sugar if it happens.

4. **Fear of failure**

Let's be clear: taking insulin does NOT mean you've failed at taking care of type 2 diabetes. Insulin is just one more tool that can be used to manage blood sugars. There's no shame in it. If your A1c is above 7 and it's not well-controlled using two different diabetes medications, starting insulin is a reasonable choice. What's not reasonable? Letting your blood sugar run out of control because you're afraid of insulin.

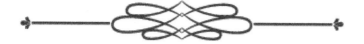

Day 19 Action Items

1. If your healthcare provider has suggested that you need insulin, but you're not yet using it, think about your fears. What's holding you back from using insulin if you need it? Do you need any more information to make a good decision about whether or not insulin is right for you?

2. Walk at an easy pace for 25-30 minutes, then stretch for 2 minutes.

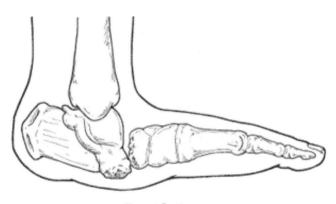

Charcot Foot

Chapter Twenty

Foot Pain and Diabetes

DIABETES FOOT PAIN CAN be long-term and life-altering. You've probably heard it said before that "when your feet are sore, you're sore all over." Several years ago, I had minor surgery on both feet at the same time, and I know first-hand that the expression springs from the truth. Here's what you need to know about how can you avoid foot pain if you have diabetes.

Causes of diabetes foot pain

Diabetes foot pain is most often caused by peripheral neuropathy: damage to the nerves in the feet. Nerves are damaged when blood sugar levels run too high. The longer your blood glucose levels are out of range, the more likely you are to experience neuropathy as well as other complications of diabetes.

How to prevent diabetes foot pain

• Keep your blood glucose levels in good control.

• Wear well-fitting shoes that don't rub or blister your feet. If you have Medicare, you may qualify for a new pair of diabetic shoes every year with a doctor's prescription. Diabetic shoes are specially designed to prevent blisters and irritation that cause diabetes foot pain.

• Consider diabetic socks made without seams that might irritate your feet.

• Check your feet every night. Look for redness, swelling, cuts, or bruises. If you're not flexible enough to look at the bottom of your feet, use a hand-held mirror to do the job, or ask a family member to check your feet for you.

• If you find a cut, redness, swelling, etc. when you check your feet and you don't see improvement within three days, call your doctor or podiatrist.

• Use a good quality moisturizer to prevent cracks in your feet.

What if I already have diabetes foot pain?

Don't beat yourself up. You can't go backward, but you can prevent any further damage to your feet by keeping your blood sugar under control. It's really important for you to check your feet every night and to get well-fitting diabetic socks and shoes — you may not have full sensation in your feet and that can make you unaware that a cut or blister has formed on the bottom of your foot until you take a look at it. Be sure to call your doctor or podiatrist right away if you notice a cut that doesn't heal.

Charcot Foot

Charcot Foot can be a result of diabetic neuropathy. When people lose lots of sensation in their feet, the bones of the foot can weaken and break. But, the person with little or no sensation doesn't feel any pain, so they keep walking. The joints in the foot can collapse and the foot takes on a "rocker bottom" shape. Charcot Foot may or may not require surgery, depending on how early it's detected. It's one reason why daily foot checks are so important for people with diabetes.

One More Thing...

I know that checking your feet is one more thing in a long list of things you're "supposed to do" to take care of your diabetes. After counting carbs and checking your blood sugar all day, most people just want to relax for a few minutes, and go to bed, already! I get it, I really do.

But...I worked in a hospital with a wound clinic for several years. When my hospital first opened the wound clinic, I was young and naive. I was envisioning gunshot wounds, and I couldn't imagine that my small town really needed that service. Then I figured out that the majority of patients in that clinic had diabetic foot ulcers. Today, I've seen more diabetic foot ulcers than I care to count. I've heard too many patients say, "I knew I was supposed to look at my feet, but I just never did it." So, please, don't be that person. Check your feet and stay out of the wound clinic.

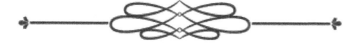

Day 20 Action Items

1. Inspect your feet. Look for redness, swelling, cuts, or bruises. Also, check to make sure that your feet don't feel warmer than the rest of your body (that's a sign of infection).

2. Find a way to make checking your feet a habit. Write it on your calendar, leave your mirror in your recliner, or set a timer on your watch or smartphone.

3. If you have trouble viewing the bottom of your feet, find a family member or a hand-held mirror to help you do the job.

4. Moisturize your feet every night to prevent cracks.

5. Consider diabetic socks if you don't have some already.

6. Consider diabetic shoes. Medicare will cover these with a prescription.

7. Walk at a brisk pace for 10 minutes, stretch for 2 minutes, then walk at an easy pace for 15 minutes.

Chapter Twenty-One

Food Pushers and Food Police

IF YOU'RE A PEOPLE-PLEASER, you may have a hard time trying to refuse food.

I was just talking with a client recently. Sadly, his brother passed away unexpectedly. Friends and relatives brought "at least 500 pounds" of food to my client's home. The food was piled up all over the kitchen and dining room and threatening to take over the rest of the house, too. One kind-hearted lady even brought a gallon jug of gravy!

My client's blood sugars had been in good control, but things got messy in the week after his brother's death. He was tempted by the treats coming into his house. Even if he had just finished eating, he felt obligated to try a little bit of every dish that was brought in so that the person who brought it would know how much he appreciated their efforts.

My client's situation was temporary. After a couple of weeks, friends and neighbors stopped bringing so many goodies. His food supply returned to normal, and so did his blood sugars. But some people live with other people who constantly encourage them to eat.

Food pushers and food police

Some of us have long-term struggles with feeling obligated to eat even when we're not hungry. We live or work with what I call "food pushers." These are people who think they know our appetites better than we do. They like to tell us when and what to eat, and they're certain we can't possibly be full yet.

The opposite of the "food pushers" are the "food police." These are the people who like to tell us when we've had enough to eat, that we need to stop, and that surely we must be full by now. These kinds of comments make some of us want to eat more just to prove the food police wrong. Ha! I'll show you...I can eat more food, a lot more food, and I'll do it right now!

The truth is, I can't look at you and know whether or not you're hungry. Likewise, you can't look at me and know whether or not I'm full. We can make an educated guess if we know how long it's been since the other person's last meal, but we really don't know anything for sure because we don't live inside anyone else's body.

Only you can decide how much food you need

You're the only one who can decide when you're hungry or full, so don't let anyone else dictate that for you. Giving someone else control over your appetite is a recipe for an unhappy gut, a weight management problem, and a potential eating disorder.

How to refuse food politely

Never argue with food pushers or food police. When you do, you invite them to believe that they have a say-so in your eating choices. It's best to acknowledge their comments in the most non-committal way possible.

Some words to use to politely refuse food:

- "You might be right." You're not saying the food pusher is right, just that they might be right. Then, you can carry on with your business as if nothing was said. For example, if your sister says, "You need to have some of this triple chocolate marshmallow fudge sauce." You can say, "You might be right" and keep eating what's on your plate without making a move toward the fudge sauce. ("You might be right" is a magic phrase that works in a lot of situations, food-wise and otherwise.)

- "I might come back for that." You might come back for that, and then again you might not. Only you will determine what you'll come back for, and that's as it should be.

- "I think I'm satisfied." Repeat as many times as needed.

Notice that neither of these phrases has anything to do with your blood sugar or your weight. You may not always want to share that you have diabetes, and your weight is really nobody's business but your own. To bring up a health condition invites discussion (and more advice), and I think to bring up weight is unnecessary. People come in all shapes and sizes and should be able to eat when they're hungry and stop when they're full without judgment from others.

It takes practice to politely refuse food

The next time someone tries to push food on you, try using one or all of the phrases above. The point is not to argue with the food pusher or food police, but to acknowledge their statement without fully agreeing with it and without changing your eating behavior. You may not feel like your efforts are successful at first, but over time, you'll become more and more comfortable with the idea that you, and only you, are in charge of what you eat.

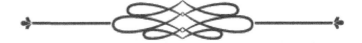

Action Items Day 21

1. Is there a "food pusher" in your life?

2. If so, think about why you may have allowed that person to dictate what you eat. Are you an adult child still listening to a parent? Has it been easier to "go along to get along?" Would you rather harm your health than hurt someone else's feelings?

3. If saying "No" to food is a sticking point for you, write out 3 polite but firm sentences you can use the next time you need to refuse food. Put them on index cards or sticky notes. Practice them in the mirror every morning until they easily roll off your tongue.

4. Rest up if you need it, or try a new activity: Salsa dancing, Zumba, yoga...the choice is yours!

Chapter Twenty-Two

Maybe It's What's Eating You

What's Eating You?

YESTERDAY, I HAD OVEN-FRIED chicken, mashed potatoes, and broccoli for dinner. I should have been satisfied. Calorie-wise, there was no way that I should have been hungry after dinner.

I took a book out to the hammock in my back yard and I tried to read. It's a good book, a psychological thriller — my favorite kind — but my mind kept wandering. My mind wandered to deciding whether to rent office space or work virtually. Then my mind wandered to the fresh oatmeal cookies sitting on the counter in my kitchen. I turned my attention back to my book, and my mind wandered to the $6000 quote I received from the orthodontist for my 7th grader. Then my mind wandered to the carton of ice cream in my freezer.

I felt stressed, and I wanted to eat to soothe my emotions. Ice cream seemed like a good plan. I went into the kitchen and got out a coffee cup. (Coffee cups keep me from eating the whole carton.) My 7th grader doesn't use coffee cups for ice cream to keep him from eating the whole carton, so I had to be satisfied with the 2 teaspoons he left in the box... and I was. I wasn't hungry to begin with. I just wanted to soothe my nerves.

My emotional eating story

When I was a little girl, my dad worked varying shifts. If he was at home at night, and if my sister and I had been "good," he would give us each a big bowl of ice cream. It was a reward for good behavior and it was also his way of showing us that he loved us. Those bowls of ice cream made me feel that all was right in my little world. Ice cream still makes me feel like all is right in the world today, if only for the few minutes I'm eating it. It's delicious, but I don't crave it for its sweet flavor, I crave it for the way it makes me feel.

The definition of emotional eating

Emotional eating is defined as "eating in response to something other than hunger." It's a form of disordered eating, although it can be mild compared to other eating disorders like anorexia and bulimia.

How to stop emotional eating

You can't change what you don't acknowledge, so the first step to stop emotional eating is to realize that it's happening to you. I like to use the Food and Mood Journal to help clients uncover emotional eating.

Use the Food and Mood Journal to Discover Emotional Eating

If you've been reading this book's chapters in order, you created a Food and Mood Journal several days ago. Take a look at your Food and Mood Journal to try to uncover any patterns:

1. Circle any times when you rated yourself as a "1" on the hunger scale, meaning you were extremely hungry.

2. Circle any times when you rated yourself as a "5" on the hunger scale, meaning you were uncomfortably full.

3. Find a highlighter and highlight any emotions you listed in your journal; happy, sad, angry, etc.

4. Find a different colored highlighter and highlight any locations you listed in your journal: home, work, restaurant, a relative's house, etc.

5. What patterns can you see?

6. Are you always a "1" at work, meaning you don't have time to eat there?

7. Do you frequently end up as a "5" at your brother's house? If so, why? Is he a food pusher to whom you haven't yet learned to say "No?"

8. Do you overeat when you're angry, or happy, or sad?

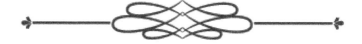

Action Items Day 22

1. If you haven't been using your Food and Mood Journal, it's not too late!

2. Look for patterns in your Food and Mood Journal as described above.

3. If you found a pattern, decide on just one small thing you'd like to do differently to change your emotional eating pattern. Make the teeny tiniest change you can make; something that is definitely doable so you'll be successful. After you make that change, you'll feel a sense of accomplishment, and then you can make another one.

4. Walk at an easy pace for 25-30 minutes.

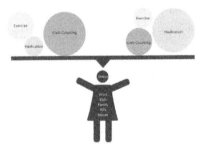

Chapter Twenty-Three

Barstools and Blood Sugars

IMAGINE SITTING ON A barstool. What if someone cut off one of the legs? Would you still want to sit on the stool? Probably not. The stool would be off-balance, and you'd come tumbling down, possibly injuring yourself in the process.

Treatment for type 2 diabetes requires a 3-pronged approach

A three-legged stool is nice and stable. If one of the legs is shorter than the other, the barstool becomes wobbly. If one leg is missing, the whole thing falls apart. Like the barstool, type 2 diabetes needs a three-pronged approach to stay in balance, too. The three "legs" used to manage type 2 diabetes are:

- Carb counting
- Physical activity
- Medication (for some people, but not all)

If we cut one of those "legs" short, blood sugar management gets wobbly. If you have diabetes and you count carbs and take your medication, but you don't exercise, you're missing out on the blood sugar-stabilizing effect of regular physical activity. You've got a wobbly barstool.

There are times when exercise isn't possible. For some people, physical limitations make exercise impossible all of the time. For those times and those people, either carbohydrate intake has to be decreased and/or medication has to be increased to keep blood sugar in check.

There are times when you'll eat more carbs than usual. At those times, you'll need to increase your physical activity and/or increase your medication (with your doctor's advice) to keep your blood sugar in range.

 The picture on your left might help illustrate how the 3 prongs of diabetes management work together [1]:

Treatment of type 2 diabetes requires flexibility

Blood sugar levels fluctuate constantly. Just when you think you've got it right, along comes a virus or a stressful deadline or even a picnic to get your blood sugar out of whack. Knowing that it's normal for your numbers to go up and down will help you keep your cool when it does happen. Which leg (or two) of your stool do you need to adjust to get back in balance?

Medication can be a lifesaver in the treatment of type 2 diabetes

I have a lot of patients who feel guilty and ashamed of themselves when they need to take medication to control their diabetes. Do you feel that way? If you do, would you feel that same guilt and shame if you needed medication for gout or arthritis? I'm guessing you wouldn't. Let go of the guilt — it's not serving anyone, especially you.

If you're waiting for your blood sugars to improve "when you get the weight off" or "when you start exercising," stop waiting. Damage to your eyes and kidneys is happening right now while you wait. If this is a particularly stressful time in your life and you know that you just can't start to exercise or change your eating plan right now, tell your doctor just that. Be blunt, and use the words, "I'm not able to change my lifestyle right now. I think it would be better if I started on a medication."

I'm a Registered Dietitian Nutritionist and a Certified Diabetes Care and Education Specialist. I'm all for changing your eating and exercise habits, but...my goal is to help you manage your blood sugars, not to shame you into starving yourself or taking up triathlons. What I want most is to prevent you from losing your vision or needing dialysis in the future. The worst thing you can do is go another year between check-ups with your blood sugar out of control while you lose vision and kidney function. There's no shame in doing what you need to do to take care of yourself, including talking with your healthcare provider about medication.

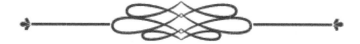

Action Items Day 23

1. Think about the "three-legged stool" of managing type 2 diabetes.

o Eating plan

o Physical Activity

o Medication

2. Is your stool balanced, or is one leg "shorter" than the others? Maybe you have an eating plan, but you're not following it. Do you forget to take your medicine more often than not? Do you have every intention of exercising in the evening, but just never get around to doing it?

3. If your "stool" has a short leg, write down your very specific plan for lengthening it. For example, if you have trouble remembering your medicine because it's not in a convenient location, you could write something like this: "I will leave my medicine beside my toothbrush so I will see it and take my medicine when I brush my teeth." Great job — now put your words into action!

4. Walk at an easy pace for 15-20 minutes. Then, alternate between "power walking" for 30 seconds and "easy walking" for 1 minute, a total of 4-6 times. After that, walk at an easy pace for another 3-5 minutes.

---

1. Credit to Megrette Fletcher M.Ed., RDN, CDCES at Weight Neutral for Diabetes Care for the concept in this diagram.

Chapter Twenty-Four

Five Appointments to Schedule ASAP

DOES THE THOUGHT OF scheduling diabetes check-ups make you want to chuck your phone in the trash? I don't know about you, but my calendar is out of control, and I don't want to make any more appointments. There's my work schedule, my son's school schedule, vet appointments for my two little dogs, eye appointments and dental appointments...the list goes on. I don't want to add another thing to my schedule, and I know you probably don't either.

I don't have diabetes, but I do have migraines. If I miss a check-up, I run out of the medication that prevents them, and then it gets really ugly. I end up losing a lot more time to headaches than I would have lost by going to the doctor.

I know your calendar is probably full, and I know that getting your diabetes check-up is not likely your idea of a good time. But...I also know that getting your diabetes check-up will save you a ton of time, money, and trouble in the long run. If you have diabetes, you need a team of experts to help you stay healthy.

These are the five most important check-ups you need to schedule every year to make sure you're on track with taking great care of your diabetes:

Your annual physical exam

Schedule a checkup with your family physician, internist, or mid-level provider (physician assistant or nurse practitioner). This person serves as your primary care provider (PCP). He or she can help you coordinate your healthcare with specialists. Your PCP can also order labs or other tests that need to happen on an annual basis, like your hemoglobin A1c.

If you have health insurance, the Affordable Care Act allows for a yearly checkup with your primary doctor at no cost.

If you've had Medicare Part B for more than a year, you can get an annual "Wellness" exam once every 12 months. The Part B deductible does not apply to the Wellness exam, so there should be no cost to you.

Your eye exam

An eye exam is recommended every year for anyone with diabetes. Your eye doctor isn't just checking to see if you need glasses. He or she is checking for diabetic retinopathy, which is damage to your eyes from poorly controlled blood sugars. Medicare will cover an annual eye exam every 12 months if you have diabetes.

A foot exam

Your primary care provider may do a foot exam during your annual checkup. If not, you'll need to see a podiatrist for a foot exam every year. A foot exam includes a visual inspection of your feet as well as the use of a monofilament — a very thin, flexible probe that your doctor will touch to different parts of your skin. This painless process is used to make sure that you have adequate sensation in your feet.

Nutrition counseling

Your Registered Dietitian Nutritionist (RDN) will help you adjust your eating plan to make sure that your blood sugars stay in range. Most private insurance companies cover Medical Nutrition Therapy (MNT), which is the name of the service provided by a Registered Dietitian Nutritionist.

Medicare covers three hours of MNT initially and two more hours every year after that. Medical Nutrition Therapy is fully covered under Medicare; there is **no** 20% copay.

Diabetes Self Management Education & Support (DSMES)

DSMES is a program that teaches people with diabetes what they need to know to stay in control of their health. I think of it as "Diabetes School". You can take DSMES classes in-person or online. The first year, DSMES consists of ten hours of class. Every year after that, Medicare recipients qualify for an additional two hours of DSMES, and most private insurance carriers cover at least two hours of DSMES as well.

Does this list seem overwhelming? Don't worry, you've got all year to spread out your appointments. You'll be well on your way to staying well in no time at all.

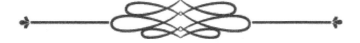

Action Items Day 24

1. Get out your calendar and write down the days when you plan to call the healthcare providers above to make appointments. You don't have to make the calls today, just make a solid plan to do it! (If you need a recommendation for a specialist, ask your primary healthcare provider.)

1. Time to mix it up again: instead of walking, dance, rake leaves, ride a bike or do any other activity that gets your heart rate up for 20-30 minutes.

Chapter Twenty-Five

Traveling with Diabetes

DELAYED FLIGHTS AND ROAD construction can be a lot to handle when you're feeling great. Add the extra burden of managing diabetes on top of that, and travel can almost be too much. Keep your cool when you travel with diabetes by taking note of these tips:

Stay hydrated

Air travel, in particular, is dehydrating. Dehydration can raise the concentration of glucose in your blood. Take extra care to drink plenty of water and other sugar-free fluids while traveling. Avoid caffeine as much as possible.

Keep your glucometer handy

If you don't usually have extreme blood sugars, you might be tempted to leave your meter at home when you travel. But you never know when you'll need to check, so pack that glucometer anyway. It's also a good idea to take the phone number for your primary care physician and your endocrinologist with you on your trip.

Pack extra diabetes medication for your trip

When traveling internationally, you must keep medicines in their original containers with their prescription labels attached. Per TSA, retaining the original packaging is not required for domestic travel, but individual states have different rules. Check ahead of time with your destination state to find out whether you need to keep medication in its original packaging. When traveling with insulin on planes, check with your airline carrier about limits on liquid medications on flights.

The best diabetes travel case for keeping insulin safe

For travel, I love Frio Insulin Cooling Wallets. They're designed to keep insulin pens or vials cool for 48 hours, and they're activated with plain water. They're lightweight, portable, and reusable, and inexpensive — a lot cheaper than losing a vial of insulin to heat! (You can find them on my Resources page if you'd like to take a look.)

Maintain your fitness routine when you travel

If you take care of your body's need for exercise, your blood glucose will be in much better control during your travels. Pack your sneakers and commit to catching up with a loved one during a walk. Fitness bands are lightweight and portable, and an excellent way to keep up a strength training routine at home and on the go.

Keep counting carbs when you travel

Unfortunately, diabetes travels with you. It's really tempting to take a vacation from carb counting, but you'll probably wind up feeling badly on vacation when your blood sugar gets out of whack. Make self-care a priority no matter where you are in the world.

The stress of travel may increase your blood sugar

A stressful travel schedule can wreak havoc on your blood sugar control. Alternatively, a hectic travel schedule with missed meals may cause blood sugar to go low. It's a good idea to wear a bracelet or another form of ID that lets people know you may need care for diabetes. If you're traveling with others, make them aware of your condition, as well as the location of your blood glucose monitor and other supplies for managing your diabetes.

Traveling with diabetes can definitely be stressful, but having your meter and plenty of supplies with you means you'll have one less thing to worry about on your adventure.

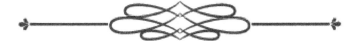

Action Items Day 25

1. Think about any upcoming travel plans.

2. Do you have the supplies you need? If not, order what you need for your next trip today.

3. Walk at an easy pace for 30-35 minutes. Stretch for 2 minutes.

Chapter Twenty-Six

Saving Money on Diabetes Supplies

HAVE YOU EVER WISHED that free diabetes supplies would fall out of the sky? It's no secret that the cost of healthcare, and especially the cost of insulin, is skyrocketing. People are skipping tests, re-using needles, and under-dosing themselves with insulin because they can't make ends meet. That makes me pretty upset, and I want to help you access any cheap or free diabetes supplies you can.

How to not to overpay for diabetes supplies

Did you know that there are "discount" diabetes supply websites that offer affiliate income to people like me, who can steer patients like you to those sites? (Affiliate income is money earned from referring a customer to a company or service. When that customer makes a purchase, the "affiliate" gets paid a fee or a percentage of the customer's purchase price — kind of like a kickback.)

Before I wrote this chapter, I checked out those "discount" sites that offer affiliate income. Guess what? I compared the price of one common type of testing strips at several of those "discount" sites to the price of the same type of testing strips at Walmart, and Walmart won every time. So, I can't recommend any of those "discount" websites. They are paying anywhere from 6-30% to people who refer buyers to them, and the person who's actually footing the bill is you.

Not every "discount" diabetes supply company has an affiliate program, but if you're curious, a quick Google search will show you which ones do.

How to find cheap and free diabetes supplies if you have Medicare or

private insurance

I'm amazed that so many of my clients don't realize that Medicare and private insurance companies cover diabetes testing supplies with a doctor's prescription. If you're in that group, you're about to save some money!

In order for Medicare to cover your supplies, your prescription must spell out all of these things:

- Whether or not you have diabetes

- What type of blood glucose monitor you need. (If you need a special talking meter because you have poor vision, the prescription needs to say that.)

- Whether or not you use insulin

- How often you should check your blood sugar

- How many test strips and lancets you need to last a month

You can get your diabetes testing supplies at a local pharmacy or through a Durable Medical Equipment (DME) company. Medicare has a rule that says you have to ask for refills, so your pharmacy or DME company can't just automatically send you supplies at the beginning of every month. Make a note to call your supplier about a week before you run out of supplies.

Best cheap diabetes supplies and meters if you're uninsured

1. The Walmart ReliOn meter isn't free, but it is inexpensive. ReliOn is consistently the least expensive meter and strips that you can buy at a store, and it's been my experience that it's just as accurate as a name-brand meter. As I'm writing this, the meter itself is $14, and a box of 25 strips is also $9.

2. If you check only once a day, you can get a free meter and lancing device plus enough strips and lancets to last you for 3 months from KnowCopay. The cost is $19.99 (Other prices available depending on how often you test.) That's cheaper than ReliOn. This is an internet/mail-order only company.

3. If you have trouble with your vision, the Prodigy meter is relatively inexpensive

(under $20) and speaks to you in four different languages so you can hear your blood glucose level instead of trying to see it. The prodigy strips are approximately $10 for a box of 50.

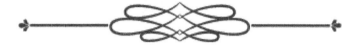

Action Steps Day 26

1. Add up all the money you spend on taking care of diabetes each month. Are you taking advantage of insurance coverage for your strips and lancets?

2. Call your doctor for a prescription if you need one.

3. If you don't have insurance coverage for supplies, investigate the three lower-cost meters above and decide if you'd like to switch the next time you run out of strips.

4. Walk at an easy pace for 25-30 minutes and then stretch for 2 minutes.

Chapter Twenty-Seven

How to Save Money on Diabetes Medications

THE COST OF DIABETES medications can be pretty inexpensive, or it can be outrageously high. Your cost depends on your insurance plan (or lack thereof) as well as what kind of medication your doctor prescribes for you. If money's tight, it's worth taking a look at your current medication list. You might be able to save a few dollars by switching things up.

If you have insurance, the cost of your diabetes medications depends on your formulary

A formulary is a list of medications that your insurance plan prefers. You get rewarded for using those medications by paying less for them. If you have health insurance or a

Medicare Advantage plan, you most likely have a formulary. You can save a great deal of money by using the medications on the formulary instead of those that are not. Take your list of preferred medications with you each time you go to the doctor so that your doctor can choose from the lowest cost "Tier I" drugs whenever possible.

To save money on the cost of diabetes medication, maximize the dose of one medication before you add another one

Sometimes patients are taking less than the maximum dose of one diabetes medication before their physician adds a second diabetes medication. That may be completely necessary in order to get your blood sugars where you want them, but then again, it may not. For example, metformin is almost always the first drug prescribed for type 2 diabetes, and the maximum dose of metformin is 2500 mg per day. Adding a second type of medication before you maximize your dose of metformin means you're going to end up with two co-pays.

If your doctor recommends adding another medication to your diabetes regimen, ask them, "Am I already on the maximum dose of my current diabetes medications?" If not, ask your doctor if they might consider trying the maximum dose first before adding a second medication. Your cost for one medication will be lower than your cost for two.

Use combination drugs to lower the cost of diabetes medication

Diabetes medications come in a single form and in combination. For example, metformin and Januvia each come as a single-drug medication. They also come in a combination called Januvamet. If your doctor were to prescribe them separately, you would pay two different copays, one for the metformin, and one for the Januvia. If your doctor were to prescribe Januvamet (both medications in one pill), you would only have to pay one copay, saving you money. As a bonus, you would also only have to remember to take one pill.

Ask for generic medications

Generic medications are cheaper, and that's the bottom line. Not to say it never happens, but I've been working in diabetes for more than twenty years, and I've never had a patient who had better blood sugars on a name-brand medication when compared to a generic.

Split pills to save on the cost of medication

Ask your doctor if it's possible to prescribe a larger amount than you take at one time and use a pill splitter to divide your pills in half. For example, you could split 1000 mg of metformin into two 500 mg doses. But...do not split pills for extended-release medications, including extended released metformin (Glucophage XR). This will destroy the coating that makes the pill extended-release.

Get your medications at a Federally Qualified Health Center

A federally qualified health center (FQHC) is a non-profit organization that provides healthcare regardless of a person's ability to pay. FQHCs also participate in the government's 340B discount drug program, which means they get medications at deeply discounted prices, and they pass those discounts on to their patients. Find an FQHC here: https://findahealthcenter.hrsa.gov/

Take advantage of Pharmaceutical Assistance Programs:

1. Search a database of pharmaceutical assistance programs for Medicare participants at Medicare.gov/plan-compare/

2. Use the Medicine Assistance Tool at https://medicineassistancetool.org/

3. Try RxAssist.org

4. NeedyMeds.org is a searchable database of patient assistance programs.

5. GoodRx.com has an online program where you can search the best prices on medications, as well as a discount card you can use at your local pharmacy. I can vouch for the card myself — it saved me quite a bit of money on a prescription.

6. There are a number of similar sites, so if you need help accessing medication, don't hesitate to ask for assistance.

It takes work to save money on diabetes medications, but if the cost of your diabetes drugs is out of control, you owe it to yourself to find a solution you can afford. Stressing out about how to pay for your medications will raise your blood sugar, and we definitely don't want that.

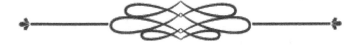

Day 27 Action Items:

1. Take a look at how much money you spend on diabetes medications alone. Is it reasonable, or is it out of control?

2. Write down a list of questions for your doctor or pharmacist about your medications. Maybe you want to ask if you're taking the maximum dose or if any of your medications come in combination.

3. If you don't have health insurance, take a look at at least one of the programs above and see if you can find a better deal on your medications.

4. Rest up! No walking today.

Chapter Twenty-Eight

How to Save Money on Insulin

I'M SHOCKED AND AMAZED at the price of insulin. According to the American Diabetes Association, the average price of insulin nearly tripled between 2002 and 2013. If you have trouble affording your insulin, you're not alone. Almost every day, a patient tells me that they have to decide between purchasing their insulin and purchasing other basic necessities.

If you use insulin, I want to help you figure out how to get the best blood sugar levels you can while keeping the cost of your insulin as low as possible. Here are four ways to save on the price of insulin:

Use human insulin instead of analog insulin

There are two main types of insulin on the market. One is human, and the other is analog. Human insulin is available in three basic varieties:

- Regular
- NPH (intermediate-acting)
- A mix of Regular and NPH, such as 70/30

Analog insulin is newer and available in an array of choices, including these:

- Short-acting (Fiasp, Humalog, Novolog, Apidra, Lispro)
- Long-acting (Lantus, Levimir, Tresiba, Basaglar, Tujeo)

Human insulin is significantly cheaper than analog insulin. It's also less flexible. Regular insulin requires that you dose yourself 20-30 minutes before you eat a meal, unlike the short-acting analogs that allow you to inject immediately before you eat.

If you're a very organized, regimented person who plans ahead, you may be OK with using Regular and NPH insulin to cut costs. If you like more freedom and flexibility in your meal schedule, then a combination of short and long-acting insulin is probably the right choice for you. Think of using Regular and NPH like driving a very basic car — perfectly safe and reliable, but not the Cadillac-level comfort and flexibility you can get with analog insulin.

Use the preferred insulin on your insurance plan's formulary

A formulary is a list of medications that your insurance plan prefers. You get rewarded for using those medications by paying less for them. If you have health insurance or a Medicare Advantage plan, you most likely have a formulary.

You can save a great deal of money by using the insulin on the formulary instead of the insulin that's not. On rare occasions, a person may be allergic to one brand of insulin or another, but for most people, one short-acting (or long-acting) insulin works just as well as the next.

Consider generic insulin

Eli Lilly makes a generic Humalog called Lispro. Take a look at their Insulin Value Program, where you may be able to fill your insulin prescription for $35 a month.

Walmart sells its own ReliOn brand of Regular and NPH (as well as 70/30) insulin for $25 per vial. You don't need a prescription, but you do need to ask for it because it's stored behind the counter. Keep in mind that this is the "older" type of human insulin, not an insulin analog. If you've been on a rapid or short-acting insulin, you'll need to make some adjustments before making the switch. Talk to your healthcare provider and Certified Diabetes Care and Education Specialist before you do that.

Take advantage of manufacturer's programs

These manufacturers have discount programs available for people without health insurance and at certain income levels:

- Lilly Diabetes Solution Center 833-808-1234

- NovoNordisk NovoCare 1-844-668-6463

- Sanofi Savings Program 1-855-984-6302

If the price of insulin is breaking your budget, talk to your healthcare team about your options. No person with diabetes should have to choose between taking care of their blood sugars and taking care of their family.

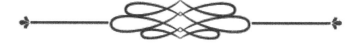

Action Steps Day 28:

1. If you take insulin, consider its cost. Is your insulin affordable?

2. Use the phone numbers and links above to investigate your options.

3. Call your diabetes educator or pharmacist and schedule a time to talk about the cost of insulin and other diabetes medications. Take your formulary with you if you have health insurance. If you want to use a

manufacturer's discount program, take that paperwork with you as well.

4. Walk at an easy pace for 25-35 minutes.

Chapter Twenty-Nine

How to Find Help for Diabetes

IF YOUR DIABETES FEELS out of control, it's time to call in a pro. There's absolutely no shame in saying "I need to get help for diabetes." In fact, reaching out for help is the smart thing to do.

So many people feel ashamed of having type 2 diabetes, and they avoid getting the help they need. But diabetes is a chronic health condition just like any other, and there is no reason to feel like it's your fault. (Yes, I know... if you weighed less, and if you exercised more...but you are where you are right now.)

If you were diagnosed with arthritis or gallstones, you'd never blame yourself. There would be no guilt or shame. So, if you're still holding onto guilt or shame about diabetes, let that go, too, and let's move on to getting the help you need.

Find a primary healthcare provider you like and trust

Ninety percent of people with diabetes are managed by general physicians, including family medicine doctors, internists, nurse practitioners, and physician assistants. All of these types of healthcare providers are qualified to manage most cases of type 2 diabetes. If you don't have a primary healthcare provider that you like and trust, you need one.

Get help for prediabetes at a Diabetes Prevention Program

Diabetes Prevention Programs (DPPs) are year-long programs that use an approved set of lessons. DPPs are designed to help people exercise at least 150 minutes each week and lose at least five percent of their body weight. The reason DPP programs have these specific goals is that research has shown that those two things are enough to prevent people with prediabetes from moving into active diabetes. Diabetes Prevention Programs are available in-person and online. Medicare and private insurance will cover DPP services, and many health departments offer these programs at no charge. **Find a DPP program here: https://www.cdc.gov/diabetes/prevention/find -a-program.html**

Participate in a Diabetes Self-Management Education and Support Program

Diabetes Self-Management Education and Support (DSMES) is a ten-hour program designed to teach people with diabetes what they need to know to take care of themselves. The program touches on everything from carb counting to medications to stress management.

DSMES programs can be in-person or virtual, and they are structured differently at different sites. For example, one program might offer ten one-hour sessions for ten weeks in a row, and another program might offer one full-day ten-hour class on

Saturdays. It's OK to find a program that fits your schedule, even if it's not local to you. (You may need to stay with a program inside of your state for insurance purposes.)

Medicare and private insurance cover DSMES. Medicare will pay for 10 hours of group DSMES the first year, and an additional 2 hours of individual DSMES every year thereafter with a healthcare provider's referral. Some health departments and Federally Qualified Health Centers provide DSMES services.

Find a DSMES program near you here: https://www.diabetes.org/diabetes/find-a-program

Get help for diabetes from a Registered Dietitian Nutritionist

If most of your diabetes questions are food-related, a Registered Dietitian Nutritionist (RDN) is your best bet. An RDN who is also a CDCES is even better.

Medicare will cover three hours of visits with an RDN the first year that you're referred for diabetes, and two hours every year after that. Medicare will also cover an additional two hours any time you have a "change in status." For example, if your A1c goes up from 7 to 9, that's a change in status that will qualify you for 2 additional hours with an RDN.

 Many private insurance companies cover visits to an RDN, and some cover unlimited visits.

Health departments and Federally Qualified Health Centers employ RDNs and may have low or no-cost options..

Find an RDN near you here: https://www.eatright.org/find-a-nutrition-expert

See a Certified Diabetes Care and Education Specialist for help with diabetes.

A Certified Diabetes Care and Education Specialist (CDCES) can be a Registered Dietitian Nutritionist, a pharmacist, a physician, a physical therapist, a physician's assistant, or a nurse. He or she must work in diabetes care for at least 1000 hours and then pass an examination that certifies him/her as competent to provide care for people with diabetes. **Find a CDCES here: https://www.cbdce.org/locate**

Get help from an endocrinologist

Endocrinologists are physicians who specialize in diabetes as well as other conditions like thyroid disease. Most people with type 2 don't see an endocrinologist, but if you feel you've tried too many things and can't get your blood sugar under control, a trip to an endocrinologist may be in order. If you want to use an insulin pump, you will likely need to see an endocrinologist for that as well. Most endocrinologists require a referral from your primary healthcare provider.

The bottom line about how to get help for diabetes

Nobody else lives in your body, and nobody else knows how you feel. If you think you need more help than you have right now, you're absolutely right. Trust your instincts when it comes to your health. Reach out for the care you need, and don't stop until you feel satisfied. You deserve to feel good about your health.

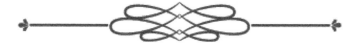

Action Steps, Day 29:

1. If you have prediabetes, consider a Diabetes Prevention Program.

2. If you have active diabetes and you've never had Diabetes Self-Management Education, find a DSMES.

3. If you need an RDN or a CDCES, that's me! See my website at www.juliecunninghamrd.com for details about my services. You can find more RDNs and CDCESs by using the **bolded web addresses** above. Keep in mind that not all RDNs specialize in diabetes, and not all CDCES are dietitians.

4. Walk at an easy pace for 10 minutes, then a brisk pace for 20 minutes, then an easy pace for 5 minutes. Stretch for 2 minutes.

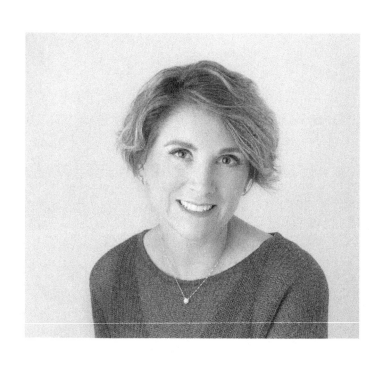

Chapter Thirty

Keep Moving Forward

YOU DID IT! You took an action towards Taming Type 2 every day for thirty days. Give yourself a giant pat on the back. You made it all the way to the end, and I'm so proud of the progress you made!

Know that diabetes is a progressive condition. If your situation changes, it's not necessarily because you did something wrong. It may be because your pancreas stopped working as well as it did before, through no fault of your own.

It' so important that you keep building on the momentum that you've built during these last thirty days, so keep adding just a few more steps to your walking plan every day, and keep taking the next tiny step towards taming type 2. Before you know it, you'll be exactly where you want to be.

If you want more help with taming type 2, find me on the web at **www.juliecunninghamrd.com**. I'd love to have you in my community!

Best wishes for a long and healthy future,

Julie

About the Author

Julie Cunningham is a Registered Dietitian Nutritionist, a Certified Diabetes Care and Education Specialist, and an International Board Certified Lactation Consultant. After earning a Bachelor of Science in Foods and Nutrition from Appalachian State University and a Master of Public Health from the University of NC at Chapel Hill, Julie began working as a Registered Dietitian in 1998.

Today, Julie makes her home with her family in Hendersonville, NC, where she owns and operates Julie Cunningham Nutrition, LLC, a nutrition practice focused on serving people with diabetes, as well as Eat, Write, Repeat, a writing service for health and wellness brands.

Acknowledgments

Thank you

Meg Stewart & Cindy Health

Made in the USA
Las Vegas, NV
17 April 2024